RENÉ
DJURUP
MD, DMSc

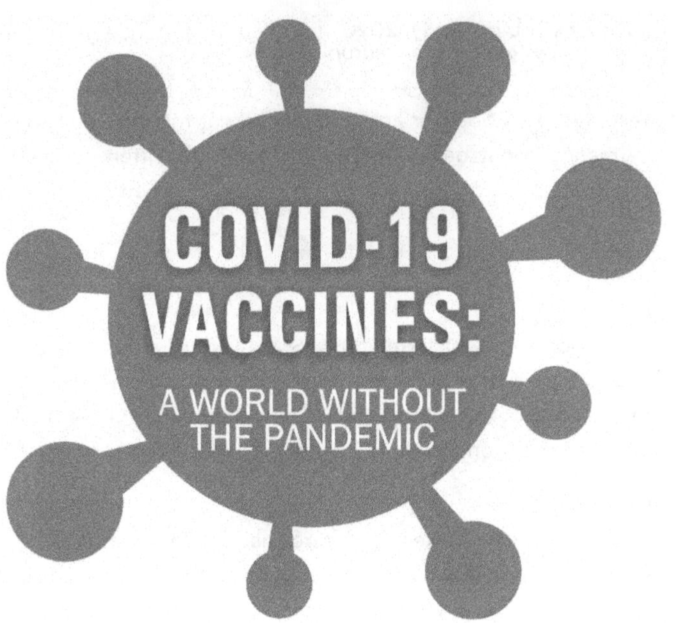

ARE THEY EVEN A POSSIBILITY?
CAN WE TRUST THESE VACCINES?
WILL THEY BE READY 2020?

Rebidu Publisher (Rebidu ApS), 2020
Copyright © 2020 by René Birger Djurup

All rights reserved. This book or any portion thereof may not be reproduced or used in any manner whatsoever without the express written permission of the author except for the use of brief quotations in a book review.

ISBN 978-87-7793-057-7

Trademarks

All terms in the book, for which Rebidu ApS is aware of a trademark claim, have been printed as suggested by the owner of the trademark. Rebidu ApS cannot warrant the accuracy of this information. Terms and names in the book are used for publication purposes only with no intention of infringement of any trademark.

Disclaimer

Every precaution has been taken to ensure that the information in the book is accurate at the time of release for printing, but the author and publisher shall have no responsibility for any errors. The information in the book is provided on an "as is" basis. Neither the author nor the publisher shall have any liability to any person or entity with respect to any loss or damage caused by or caused by information contained in the book or by use hereof by any means.

Cover images

The cover images are reproduced by permission from GoodStudio/Shutterstock.com, eamesBot/Shutterstock.com, and Bakhtiar Zein/Shutterstock.som.

Contact

To report any error in the book, please send an e-mail to rene@rebidu.com. Please state the title of the book in the subject header.

PREFACE

The COVID-19 pandemic is one of the worst disasters to affect humankind in the last century. While other infectious diseases like the flu and HIV have taken more lives, no other infectious epidemic in the last 100 years has so greatly influenced us. By the end of June 2020, more than 10 million people had been infected with the COVID-19 virus, and more than 500,000 people had died from the disease.

The rapid spread of the highly contagious COVID-19 virus and its high death toll quickly led to unprecedented global lockdowns and restrictions in people's daily lives.

Although lockdown measures have been reasonably effective, they cannot be maintained forever without causing irreparable damage to our societies and social lives. Many societies had therefore started easing their respective lockdowns. A few days later, the number of infected people per day started to increase again. This shows that it is not possible to ease the lockdowns without risking a new increase in the number of infected people— and a consequent increase in the death toll.

We therefore need to quickly build up immunity to the COVID-19 virus. This can happen in only two ways: by natural immunity following an infection with COVID-19 or by vaccination with a COVID-19 vaccine.

By natural infection with the COVID-19 virus, many people will become severely ill, and some will inevitably die. In the US, the number of deaths might exceed one million people. This would be an unacceptably high death toll. Building up population immunity by natural infection is hence not a viable way.

The alternative to building up immunity by natural infection is vaccination. Vaccines are very safe. Most likely, there would be no deaths caused by vaccination with COVID-19 vaccines. The problem is that right now, there is no COVID-19 vaccine available for mass vaccinations. The world is therefore desperately awaiting an effective vaccine against COVID-19.

An unprecedented vaccine development race has kicked off. When I finished editing this book June 24, more than 140 vaccines were being developed, and 16 of them were already being tested in humans. This gives us hope that an effective vaccine is within sight—although it may not be just around the corner.

In this book, you will learn how vaccines are developed, manufactured, and tested to ensure that any COVID-19 vaccine will actually protect the vaccinated person and not lead to any harm. You'll also learn about the 16 frontrunners in the race to bring such a vaccine to the market. We'll explore each lead candidate's likelihood of success.

After reading the book, you'll be able to judge for yourself whether it's at all realistic to expect effective COVID-19 vaccines to be freely available in 2020—and whether they can end the pandemic, open up our societies and borders, and bring our lives back to normal.

I have written this book for the general adult reader who wants to know more about COVID-19 vaccines and the likelihood that they will soon be available. The book may also be of interest to healthcare workers, journalists, analysts, and other professionals.

The book goes into some depth regarding immunology and vaccine development, but it does not assume that the reader has any previous knowledge about natural sciences. Any scientific term that's needed to comprehend a vaccine technology is explained in an easy-to-understand way.

At the end of each chapter, you'll find a list of references. I've decided not to include in-text citations in order to simplify the text and make it easier to read.

The technical editing of this book ended on June 24, 2020. This means that new COVID-19 vaccines entering testing in humans after this date are not described. However, you'll have enough knowledge to evaluate any new candidate yourself.

Last, I want to thank Isabelle Anne Abraham for her outstanding copy editing. Isabelle contributed significantly to making the book easier to read and understand. She also ensured linguistic consistency throughout the text. I had to make some last-minute changes, and so I take full responsibility for any typos, etc. I also want to thank Shabbir Hussain for his excellent book cover design.

I hope you'll enjoy reading this book as much as I enjoyed writing it.

June 30, 2020
René Djurup

TABLE OF CONTENTS

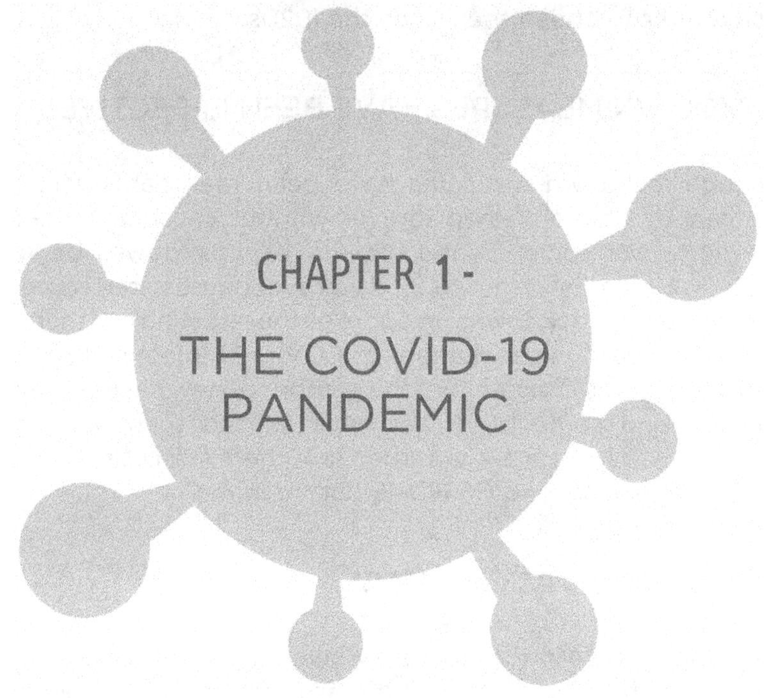

CHAPTER 1 -
THE COVID-19
PANDEMIC

The COVID-19 pandemic is one of the worst disasters to affect humankind in the last century. While other infectious diseases like the flu and HIV have taken more lives, no other infectious epidemic in the last 100 years has so greatly influenced us.

The rapid spread of the highly contagious COVID-19 virus and its high death toll quickly led to unprecedented global lockdowns and restrictions in people's daily lives. In only a couple of months, the lockdowns resulted in the loss of millions of jobs, a massive drop in business earnings, and a severe and rapid stock market crash that hasn't been seen since the 1920s.

LOCKDOWN MEASURES HAVE BEEN EFFECTIVE

Although lockdown measures have been reasonably effective, they cannot be maintained forever without causing irreparable damage to our societies and social lives. Lockdowns began in March 2020, and in June 2020, several countries started easing their respective lockdowns. In some of these countries, there has been an increase in the number of COVID-19 infections per day. The latest figures indicate that the number of new cases in several countries and some US states have started to go up again. Additionally, WHO recently warned that there still is a risk that we may be hit by a second COVID-19 outbreak.

THE COVID-19 VACCINE RACE

The world is therefore desperately awaiting an effective vaccine against the dreaded COVID-19 disease. We are in the middle of an unprecedented vaccine race. Never before have so many research institutions and pharma companies been involved in the development of a vaccine against a disease. Many smaller biotech companies have received solid funding and/or entered into profitable collaborations with big pharma companies. The massive interest in developing and manufacturing COVID-19 vaccines and the substantial financial support increase the likelihood that one of the more 140 candidates currently in development (June 24, 2020) will succeed and lead to a useful vaccine within an unprecedented brief time.

ALL KNOWN TECHNOLOGIES FOR MAKING VACCINES HAVE BEEN UTILIZED

All known vaccine technologies are being tried in order to rapidly create a safe and effective vaccine. Everyone wants to be the first to bring their COVID-19 vaccine candidate to the market. Several institutions and companies have stated that they can deliver millions of doses this year (2020) and one billion or more next year. Each day, the media reports that a new, promising, and effective vaccine is just around the corner.

GOING BEYOND THE NEWS

This book goes beyond the hype and introduces you to the world of vaccine development. You will learn how vaccines are developed, manufactured, and tested in animals and humans to ensure that any marketable COVID-19 vaccine will actually protect the vaccinated person and not lead to any harm.

We'll delve into the COVID-19 vaccine landscape, and you'll find out about each of the front-runners in the desperate race to bring such a vaccine to the market. Each lead candidate's likelihood of success will be evaluated. After reading the book, you'll be able to judge for yourself whether it's at all realistic to expect effective vaccines to be freely available in 2020—and whether they can end the COVID-19 pandemic, open up our societies and borders, and bring our lives back to normal.

THE COVID-19 PANDEMIC TIMELINE

On December 31, 2019, it was reported by Chinese authorities that a new lung disease, a type of pneumonia, had been observed in the Chinese city Wuhan. Prior to this, a few patients in Wuhan had sought medical treatment for illnesses that seemed like influenza or a common pneumonia. The testing of the patients began mid-December and indicated that they had a viral infection. Tests for influenza were negative. Some of the patients underwent an advanced X-ray evaluation (a CT scan) of the lungs. The doctors found a pattern that resembled the picture seen during the SARS epidemic of 2002–2003.

Earlier, on December 24, the doctors took a specimen of the secretion from the airways from a patient with pneumonia of an unknown cause and sent it for analysis in a lab. The result came back on December 30 and suggested that the pneumonia was caused by a SARS-like virus. Officially, the result was first considered faulty, but measures to effectively deal with a possible new virus outbreak were quickly put in place by the local Chinese health authorities in Wuhan.

On December 30, it was confirmed by another lab that the airway secretion specimen mentioned above was most likely a SARS-like virus. The local and central Chinese Center for Disease Control and Prevention (CCDC) became involved, and the local hospitals in Wuhan received instructions on how to deal with patients showing up with signs of the new virus disease.

On December 31, the Chinese public were informed about a possible outbreak of a new type of pneumonia in Wuhan. International news agencies quickly picked up the information. At this time, 27 people had been infected, seven had become seriously ill, but no one had died from the new disease. There was no indication that the disease could spread from person to person. The cause of the disease was still under investigation.

On May 10, 2020, when I started writing this book, more than four million people had been infected. The COVID-19 virus had hit more than 180 countries, and the disease had killed more than 280,000 people. When I finished editing the book (June 24), the number of infected people had increased to more than 10 million. The number of deaths had increased to more than 500,000. It took just 45 days to double the number of infected and dead.

THE WORST PANDEMIC SINCE THE SPANISH FLU

One of the worst pandemics since the Spanish Flu, which ravaged the world in 1918–1919, had hit humankind. It turned out that we were largely unprepared for such a pandemic, and despite earlier outbreaks of very similar coronavirus diseases (SARS in 2002–2003 and MERS in 2012), no effective medicine or vaccine was available.

The disease was later called COVID-19 (coronavirus disease 2019), whereas the virus was officially named SARS-CoV-2 (due to its similarity to the "original" SARS virus). The term "SARS-CoV-2" seems to be rather infrequently used in the media, and in this book, I'll use the term "COVID-19" for both the disease and the virus, except for where it could cause confusion.

LOCKDOWN AND STRINGENT HYGIENIC MEASURES

As it was recognized that the new coronavirus very quickly spread from country to country despite several safety measures—hand disinfection, wearing of masks in public spaces, curfews, closing of borders, and so on—an almost desperate race for the development of safe and effective drugs and vaccines kicked off.

The unprecedented lockdown measures turned out to be effective. The number of infected people per day has started to decrease in the countries that were the first to implement the lockdown measures or that instituted the most stringent regulations. The Johns Hopkins University in the US maintains an excellent web page (please see the references at the end of the chapter) on which we can see the number of infected people per day in many countries—inclusive of the US of course.

Regarding the US, even though the number of new cases per day has for some time been decreasing, there's still (June 19, 2020) an uptrend in 21 states. And on June 26, the highest number of infected cases in one day in the US—40,000—was reported.

Globally, the number of COVID-19 infected people continues to increase. On the day when I started editing this chapter (June 19), WHO reported that the highest number of new COVID-19 cases, 150,000, was observed on Thursday, June 18. This number was already surpassed by June 21, when more than 180,000 new cases were reported. On the same day, the US reported the biggest jump in new cases since early May. The COVID-19 virus is still a threat.

THE HOPE OF DEVELOPING HERD IMMUNITY

No one knows if or when the pandemic will end—or if it will end by itself. Some experts and authorities have relied on the development of herd immunity. Herd immunity occurs when a sufficient number of people have been infected *and* have developed immunity to an infectious organism such as the COVID-19 virus.

Herd immunity may develop as a result of either natural infections from the COVID-19 virus or vaccination with a COVID-19 vaccine. To better understand what it takes to develop herd immunity, we need to look at the reproduction number. Whereas only a few people may have heard about the reproduction number prior to the COVID-19 pandemic, the term has now entered everyday language. The reason for this is because the reproduction number is of paramount importance for the development of the pandemic. In brief, if the reproduction number is above 1.0, the pandemic will continue to infect more and more people. If it is below 1.0, it will eventually die out.

THE REPRODUCTION NUMBER R

The percentage of a population that needs to be immune to disease depends on the infectious organism's reproduction number R. The reproduction number is defined as the number of new cases for each infected person. If a person on average infects three other people, the reproduction number is said to be 3. If the reproduction number is above 1.0, the number of infected people will increase, and an epidemic or pandemic will occur or worsen. If the reproduction number is below 1.0, the number of infected people will decrease. and the epidemic will eventually die out. The reproduction number exists in two forms: R_0 and R_e. We'll look at the difference between these two numbers below. For now, we'll just call the reproduction number "R."

IF THE REPRODUCTION NUMBER IS ABOVE 1.0, THE PANDEMIC WILL CONTINUE

Let's look at an example. If the reproduction number is 3, 10 infected people will infect 30 other people, who will then infect 90 people, who will infect 270 people, and so on. After 10 rounds of infection, the 10 people originally infected will have caused the infection of 590,490 people. If an infected person infects another person within one week, the number of infected people would have grown from 10 to almost 600,000 people in just 10 weeks.

These calculations are based on a number of assumptions. Some of the more important assumptions are: There must be enough healthy people to infect, and the infected people must come quickly into contact with people who have not been infected yet. There must be no restriction of contact between people. The infected people do not die. If you are interested in how I arrived at these numbers of new cases (N) after X rounds, the formula is: N = RX.

IF THE REPRODUCTION NUMBER IS ABOVE 1.0, THE PANDEMIC WILL DIE OUT

If, on the other hand, the reproduction number is 0.3, 100,000 infected people will only infect 30,0000 people, who will again infect 10,000 people, and so on. After 10 rounds of infection, there will be less than one new person infected in the next round. The epidemic will eventually die out.

THE DIFFERENCE BETWEEN R_0 AND R_E

The reproduction number as mentioned exists in two forms: R_0 and R_e. R_e is also sometimes called R_t, and R_0 is also called the basic reproduction number. This number tells us how many people an infected person can infect in a group of people or population that has not yet developed any immunity to the infection.

When the COVID-19 virus disease started in Wuhan, the reproduction number observed before any travel restrictions and hygienic measures were implemented was the basic reproduction number R_0. R_e is the number of people in any given population who can be infected by an infected individual at any given time. It depends on a number of factors. It decreases when social distancing or curfews are implemented. It also decreases when people become immunized, either as a result of infection from the COVID-19 virus or through vaccination. If a significant percentage of the population dies, the effective reproduction number also decreases. Measures that prevent the spread of the virus, such as frequent hand disinfection or wearing face masks, will also decrease the effective reproduction number R_e.

THE REPRODUCTION NUMBER FOR THE COVID-19 DISEASE

Several estimates of the basic reproduction number R_0 have been presented. In the example above, I for simplicity set it to 3. However, most estimates center around the figure 2.6. We'll use this figure for our further evaluation. The number is not particularly high; here are some comparisons:

- For measles, it is around 14—in a population that has not been vaccinated.
- For the eradicated smallpox disease, it was around 6.
- For seasonal flu, it is around 1.3.

This means that the COVID-19 virus is about two times as infectious as seasonal flu.

COVID-19 IS MUCH MORE INFECTIOUS THAN THE FLU

If we assume that the basic reproduction number for the COVID-19 disease is 2.6—currently our best guess—then 10 people infected with COVID-19 would lead to 141,167 infected people in just 10 weeks (assuming that one round of infection takes one week).

Compare this figure with the number 590,490 that we found above, when we assumed that the reproduction number was 3. If the reproduction number is 2.6 and not 3, there will be 75% less people infected after 10 rounds. An accurate estimate of the reproduction number is therefore of paramount importance for predicting how the pandemic will evolve—but unfortunately, an accurate estimate does not exist.

For seasonal flu, the figure would be only 138 people—again, assuming that one round takes one week. As you'll learn below, the death rate for the COVID-19 virus disease is also much higher than for seasonal flu. So now, we can already with certainty say: The COVID-19 disease is not just "another flu." It is a highly infectious and highly deadly disease.

IMMUNITY THROUGH NATURAL DISEASE
OR VACCINATION

Immunity may develop through natural infection from the COVID-19 virus or through vaccination. The development of natural immunity requires that the person becomes infected. Some people do not get any symptoms at all and do not feel ill. Most infected people just get a common-cold-like infection and recover quickly. However—and this is a very important "however"—many people become severely ill. And many of those people die. Furthermore, doubt has recently been cast on the durability of the immunity following an infection with the COVID-19 virus. It may be possible that the level of protecting antibodies in patients with no or only mild symptoms will start to decrease after just a few months. Some scientists estimate that the immunity after a COVID-19 virus infection may only last 6 to 12 months.

THE COVID-19 DEATH RATE

The death rate of COVID-19 is high compared to the death rate of seasonal flu. It is difficult to say precisely how much higher the death rate of COVID-19 is, but it seems that it's at least five times as high as seasonal flu (see below).

The number of people who have died from COVID-19 in the US was 118,205 (June 20) out of the 2,172,212 who are known to have been infected. The number known to have been infected is called the confirmed cases (see below). By dividing the number of people who have died from COVID-19 by the number of confirmed cases, we'll get the case fatality rate. On June 20, 2020, it was 5.44%. As we'll see below, the case fatality rate will almost always be higher than the death rate.

CONFIRMED CASES AND INFECTED CASES

A person who is known to have been infected is called a "confirmed" case. This requires in many countries that the infection of the COVID-19 virus has been confirmed by a lab test that looks for the presence of the COVID-19 genes. It is called a PCR test, and often conducted as a mouth or nose swab.

However, many people infected with the COVID-19 virus do not get any symptoms or only get mild symptoms. They do not consult a doctor or go to a hospital. They are "infected cases" but not "confirmed cases." If a person does not feel ill, they usually won't get a test for the COVID-19 virus. There will therefore be some people who are (or who have been) infected, but for whom the infection has not been confirmed.

As long as not all people in a population are tested, the number of confirmed cases will be lower than the number of infected cases. Testing all people in a population has so far only been done in smaller isolated societies.

Early in the pandemic, it was estimated that only 1 in 12 cases in the US was confirmed. However, more recent data indicated that 1 out of 2.2 infected cases was confirmed. If only 1 out of 12 infected cases was confirmed, the death rate would "only" be about 0.45% (5.44% divided by 12) for the COVID-19 disease, but it would still be about five times higher than for seasonal flu (death rate: 0.1%). If, however, 1 out 2.2 infected cases was confirmed, the death rate would be about 2.5% (5.44% divided by 2.2). This would be 25 times as high as the death rate for seasonal flu. In any case, the death rate for the COVID-19 disease in the US and elsewhere is much higher than for seasonal flu.

NO ONE WAS IMMUNE TO THE COVID-19 DISEASE FROM THE START

Many people are immune to influenza viruses that cause seasonal flu—either due to previous infections or due to vaccinations. This means that only a small proportion of the population (usually less than 10%) is susceptible to infection from seasonal flu. In contrast, almost all people were susceptible to the COVID-19 virus when the pandemic first started. If all people (100% of the population) were susceptible, a death rate of 0.45% would mean that 1,485,000 in the US (population size approximately 330 million) could die from the COVID-19 infection.

On the one hand, this may be seen as a worst-case scenario: When a sufficient number of people has been infected (about 60%; see later in this chapter), the COVID-19 epidemic in the US would start dying out, and the death toll would be less. On the other hand, the number of confirmed cases compared to the number of infected people may have been underestimated. As we saw above, it's possible that only one out of 2.2. infected people is actually a confirmed case. This would mean that the "real" death rate could be as high as 2.5% (see also above). The death toll would then be above eight million people—if the whole population would be infected. Fortunately, this will not be the case, due to among other things the social distancing and improved hygienic measures enforced on us. As we'll explore below, only an effective vaccine can bring the pandemic to an end—and our social lives back to the normal.

THE DEATH TOLL TO ACQUIRE HERD IMMUNITY THROUGH NATURAL INFECTION IS TOO HIGH

If we assume that "only" 70% of the US population could become infected with the COVID-19 virus before the epidemic would start dying out, and that only 1 out of 12 infected cases is confirmed, it would still take about one million deaths to develop immunity. Most societies would consider such a death toll much too high to be acceptable to develop herd immunity. The real death toll would likely be much higher. We can with certainty conclude that the death toll required to develop herd immunity through natural infection would be far too high for any society.

THE BETTER PATH TO HERD IMMUNITY: VACCINATION

The only other way to increase immunity in a population is through vaccination. For other infectious diseases such as measles, vaccination has shown to be tremendously effective in making a population immune.

Even though measles is much more infectious than COVID-19 (see below), the number of new measles cases in the US per year was only 1,282 in 2019. This was the highest number in the last 10 years. In 2016, 2017, and 2018, it was 86, 120, and 375. The increase in the number of measles cases is likely due to the fact that some children are not vaccinated against measles. Still, the figures show that vaccination can almost completely prevent the outbreak of even a highly infectious disease.

> In this context, it's worth mentioning that the most dangerous of all infectious diseases, smallpox, was eradicated through effective vaccination. Smallpox had a reproduction number of 6 and a death rate of 30%. After 10 infection rounds, one infected person could (in theory) infect more than 60 million other people—and kill 30% of them (more than 18 million). Before it got to that point, smallpox would have run out of new individuals to infect, so the number of infected and dead people would be less. There are, however, reports of smallpox eradicating almost all inhabitants in villages where those inhabitants had no immunity to smallpox.

Vaccines Are Very Safe

Vaccines are very safe; they are the safest group of drugs. They *have* to be so because while other drugs are given to people who already have a disease (for example hypertension, diabetes, or cancer), vaccines are given to healthy people. Society's willingness to accept side effects, particularly severe side effects, is therefore very low. A given person will not know whether they will get the infectious disease at all and will hence be very reluctant to accept any severe side effect. However, due to the seriousness of COVID-19 and the high risk of becoming severely ill or even dying from this disease, most people would likely be willing to accept a higher risk for a COVID-19 vaccine than for some other vaccines, for example the seasonal flu vaccine.

THERE IS NO ALTERNATIVE TO VACCINATION

There is no alternative to vaccination to develop immunity to the COVID-19 virus and to prevent severe illness. Drugs that can increase the survival rate in severely ill people are becoming available. Antibodies (see Chapter 2) from patients who have recovered from a COVID-19 infection may also be used to treat patients with a severe COVID-19 illness.

Drugs and antibodies would only be used to treat severely ill patients. They will not prevent any new cases of the disease, and they will not increase any population's immunity to the COVID-19 virus. So, if we want to bring the pandemic to an end, there is no alternative to an effective COVID-19 vaccine.

THE IMMUNITY NEEDED TO END THE PANDEMIC

You may have seen various figures for the immunity needed in a population to start bringing the COVID-19 pandemic to an end. A commonly cited figure is 62%. How did scientists arrive at this figure? The short answer is that they used a formula. Before we take a look at the formula, I can reveal that the figure only depends on the COVID-19 virus reproduction number.

The basic reproduction number R_0 is often used, but I think it might be more realistic to use the effective reproduction number R_e. One reason why is because some of the good hygienic measures that have been enforced on us may stay with us for some time even after mass vaccination has begun. Frequent handwashing, avoiding handshaking, and so on will keep the effective reproduction number R_e lower than the basic reproduction number R_0. They will not only reduce the number of COVID-19 infections, but also that of many other infectious diseases such as the flu.

As mentioned, the immunity needed in a population to initiate the end of an epidemic depends on only the reproduction number. The relation between the immunity needed and reproduction number is very simple: The higher the reproduction number, the higher the number of immune people needed to bring the epidemic to an end. If we assume that the reproduction number for flu is 1.3, for COVID-19 2.6, and for measles 14, the immunity needed to prevent or end an epidemic is 23% (flu), 62% (COVID-19), and 83% (measles). For those who are interested, the formula is 1 - (1/R).

Scientists arrived at the 62% figure regarding the immunity needed to bring the epidemic to an end by using the basic reproduction number 2.6. If we can make so many people immune through vaccination, we'd no longer need any of the hygienic measures that are currently in place.

WHAT IF THE VACCINE GIVES ONLY INCOMPLETE PROTECTION?

Ideally, any COVID-19 vaccine should protect us against the COVID-19 disease for the rest of our lives. And it should prevent us from becoming infected at all. Even if these ambitious goals can't be met, a COVID-19 vaccine offering protection for only a short time—or "only" protecting us from becoming severely ill—will still be very useful.

WHAT IF THE VACCINE OFFERS ONLY SHORT-TERM PROTECTION?

A vaccine protecting all vaccinated people for one year would bring the current pandemic to an end—if all people could be vaccinated within a short time. This is a technical challenge (see Chapter 3 and 4). Revaccinations each year might be needed to maintain a reasonably high immunity, but it would still be possible to prevent major epidemics with a vaccine offering only short-term protection.

WHAT IF THE VACCINE ONLY PROTECTS US FROM BECOMING SEVERELY ILL?

A COVID-19 vaccine does not need to offer complete protection against the disease either. Ideally, it should protect us from becoming infected at all. (This is sometimes called sterilizing immunity.) However, a COVID-19 vaccine protecting us from getting infections in the lower airways and hence from becoming severely ill would still be very useful.

CAN WE DEVELOP A VACCINE AGAINST COVID-19?

Before we start exploring COVID-19 vaccines, we'll take a closer look at the COVID-19 virus. This will enable you to better understand the information that we're going to explore later.

CORONAVIRUSES AND THE COVID-19 VIRUS

COVID-19 belongs to a family of viruses. There are seven viruses in this family that can infect humans. There are many other coronaviruses in the family that can infect other mammals and birds. Often, a given coronavirus can infect more than one species. Many coronaviruses infect bats, but the bats don't get ill in the same way that we do. Apparently, the bats' immune system is capable of keeping coronaviruses, including the COVID-19 virus, at bay.

Four of the coronaviruses that can infect humans usually only cause common colds in the upper airways and are rarely dangerous. However, within the last 20 years, three dangerous types of coronaviruses have emerged: SARS (2002), MERS (2012), and COVID-19 (2019).

All coronaviruses are RNA viruses. This means that their genes are made up of RNA. In contrast, our genes consist of DNA. Coronaviruses are the largest RNA viruses known and possess a highly effective mechanism to infect human cells and take control over the human protein synthesis machinery.

The COVID-19 virus is also called SARS-CoV-2. This name shows that it is very similar to the SARS virus. Among other things, it uses the same mechanism as the SARS virus to enter our cells.

The SARS and the COVID-19 viruses both use a receptor on our cells, called the ACE2 receptor, to get into our cells. The ACE2 receptor is involved in the regulation of our blood pressure and is found in our airways and in many other organs.

The COVID-19 virus consists of a core, where the RNA genes are found, and a shell. The shell consists of proteins that among other things enables the COVID-19 virus to infect our cells. Outside the shell, the COVID-19 has an envelope that consists of fat. This explains why soap is good at removing COVID-19 from our hands and surfaces: Soap breaks down the COVID-19 envelope and makes it vulnerable to degradation.

The COVID-19 virus shell and envelope contain four proteins: The spike protein (S protein), the nucleocapsid protein (N protein), the membrane protein (M protein), and the envelope protein (E protein). The COVID-19 virus uses the S protein to enter our cells. The vaccines that we are going to hear about in later chapters mostly target the whole COVID-19 virus or its S protein (or even a smaller part thereof). When the whole COVID-19 virus is used to make a vaccine, our body may make antibodies against all four proteins, but the antibodies found in blood specimens from infected people are directed at the S protein or the N protein.

DEVELOPING VACCINES AGAINST THE COVID-19 VIRUS

The very first step in bringing a vaccine to the market is obviously to develop it. I would like to stress that the creation of a new vaccine is basically a development task. Today we already have a number of platforms on which new vaccines may be developed. This means that we do not need an invention or a breakthrough, although such terms are occasionally used by the media.

Furthermore, we didn't start from scratch when we began developing COVID-19 vaccines. Many institutions had significant experience with the development of vaccines against SARS or MERS before the COVID-19 pandemic broke out.

In the following chapters, we'll first explore the general approach to the development of a vaccine from the lab bench to the large-scale commercial manufacturing of millions and billions of doses. We'll then take a close look at each of the major platforms that are being used to develop COVID-19 vaccine candidates.

We'll start by looking into how vaccination may make us immune to infectious diseases (Chapter 2). You'll then learn how vaccines are manufactured—from the construction of the vaccine in the lab, to the production of the first few doses, to the industrial manufacturing of billions of doses (Chapter 3). In Chapter 4, we'll examine how new vaccines are tested in animals and humans before they may be approved for general use.

After this general introduction to vaccines, we'll evaluate each platform that is used for the development of COVID-19 vaccines. We'll also look at each institution, biotech company, or pharma company that's involved in the development of the COVID-19 vaccines that are already being tested in humans. Below, we'll use the term "company" for any institution, biotech company, or big pharma.

For each COVID-19 vaccine candidate that is being tested in humans (the front-runners), we'll consider the following factors:

- What is the target for the vaccine? The whole COVID-19 virus, the S protein, or another part of the COVID-19 virus?

- How is the vaccine being manufactured? Is it a known, well-established method that the company has experience with?

- Has the company previously developed other coronavirus vaccines, for example against SARS or MERS?

- How many doses of any other coronavirus vaccine against SARS or MERS has this company produced?

- Have they tested other coronavirus vaccines in animals? If so, what were the results? Did the vaccine produce neutralizing antibodies (see Chapter 2)? Did it protect the animals against the disease or against severe disease (see Chapter 3)?

- Has the company tested other coronavirus vaccines against SARS or MERS in humans? Did it produce neutralizing antibodies?

- Does the company have the needed funding—the financial strength—to develop the manufacturing process on a large scale and to carry out clinical trials in many people?

- Has the company entered into collaborations with governmental institutions (for example NIH, NIAID, HHS,

or BARDA in the US) that can support the development
and manufacturing?

- Where do we receive all this information from? Scientific
  papers (highest credibility)? Company presentations?
  Press releases? At the end of each chapter, you'll find a
  list of the more important references that I have used.

For each of the 16 COVID-19 vaccine candidates that are being
tested in humans, I've tried to include all these factors in my
evaluation of the vaccine and the likelihood that it will lead to a
safe and effective COVID-19 vaccine.

REFERENCES

Aronson, JK; Brassey, J; Mahtani, KR. 2020. ""When will it be over?": An introduction to viral reproduction numbers, R0 and Re ". CEBM, Last Modified 14 April, accessed 30 June. https://www.cebm.net/covid-19/when-will-it-be-over-an-introduction-to-viral-reproduction-numbers-r0-and-re/.

Bohk-Ewalda, C; Dudelb, C; Myrskylä,M. 2020. "A demographic scaling model for estimating the total number of COVID-19 infections." MedRxiv, Last Modified 26 May, accessed 30 June. https://www.medrxiv.org/content/10.1101/2020.04.23.20077719v3.

CDC. 2020. "Measles Cases and Outbreaks." accessed 1 July. https://www.cdc.gov/measles/cases-outbreaks.html.

European Centre for Disease Prevention and Control. 2020. "Immune responses and immunity to SARS-CoV-2." European Centre for Disease Prevention and Control, Last Modified 11 June, accessed June 30.

Johns Hopkins University. 2020. "Coronavirus Resource Center." Johns Hopkins University, Last Modified 30 June, accessed June 30. https://coronavirus.jhu.edu/.

Jr., Lovelace B. 2020. "Why a coronavirus vaccine might be ready early next year — and what could go wrong." CNBC, Last Modified 21 May, accessed 30 June.

Rettner, A. 2020. "How does the new coronavirus compare with the flu?", Last Modified 14 May, accessed 30 June. https://www.livescience.com/new-coronavirus-compare-with-flu.html.

Ritchie, H. et al. 2020. "United States: Coronavirus Pandemic." OurWorldInData.org, Last Modified 29 June, accessed 29 June. https://ourworldindata.org/coronavirus/country/united-states?country=~USA.

WHO 2020. "Draft landscape of COVID-19 candidate vaccines." WHO, Last Modified June 29, accessed 30 June. https://www.who.int/publications/m/item/draft-landscape-of-covid-19-candidate-vaccines.

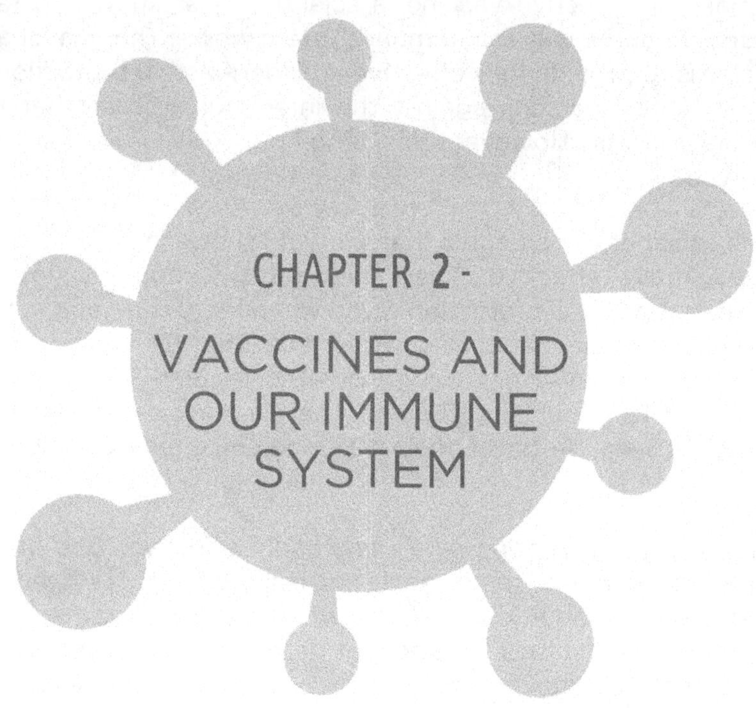
CHAPTER 2 -
VACCINES AND
OUR IMMUNE
SYSTEM

OUR IMMUNE SYSTEM

Our immune system is as highly developed as our brain. It has, over millions of years, proven highly effective in preventing and combating infectious diseases caused by many different microorganisms, including viruses. Now and then, however, it needs help from drugs or vaccines.

To make an effective vaccine, a scientist must know and take advantage of the way our immune system works. The goal of any vaccine is to provide fully effective and long-lasting protection in all vaccinated persons against the infectious disease that the vaccine targets. However, this ambitious goal is not always achieved.

Some vaccines, for example the yearly flu shot, are unfortunately only partially effective. They may offer some, but not all, vaccinated persons protection. Even when there is a good match between the circulating flu virus and the flu vaccine, the protection is only in the range of 40% to 60%. If the match between the circulating flu and the flu vaccine is less, the protection may be lower than 40%—or there may even be no benefit at all.

That said, many vaccines are remarkably effective. One of the greatest triumphs of medicine, if not the greatest, has been the complete eradication of smallpox by vaccination. Another good example is the measles vaccine that protects against measles for the rest of one's life.

To make an effective vaccine, a scientist must try to understand why some vaccines are remarkably effective, whereas others only offer partial or short-term protection. For a vaccine to be effective, it should be designed so that it takes full advantage of the different components of our immune system.

THE INNATE IMMUNE SYSTEM

Our immune system consists of many different parts or lines of defense. We all have an innate immune system that protects us from being infected and becoming ill from many infections by microorganisms—even though this immune system has never met those microorganisms before.

THE WHITE BLOOD CELLS

The innate immune system consists of many different parts, one of the more important being the white blood cells. There are many different types of white blood cells in our blood and in our tissues. Each type has its own specific function.

A fundamental feature of the innate immune system is that it recognizes microorganisms, including viruses, that it has never met before as being foreign and being invaders. It starts off an immune response against the unknown microorganisms as soon as it has detected them. Often, it succeeds on its own in eliminating the unwanted microorganisms, but it nearly always starts up the adaptive immune system, too. We'll explore this below.

THE INNATE IMMUNE SYSTEM RECOGNIZES FOREIGN PATTERNS

The innate immune system works by recognizing patterns (molecules on the surface of the microorganism) that microorganisms such as viruses possess. These patterns are not found on human cells. The innate immune system therefore immediately knows when a foreign organism tries to invade the body.

The innate immune system rarely makes headlines, except in the scientific press, but it is a highly important part of our immune defense.

MORE ABOUT THE WHITE BLOOD CELLS

It is outside the scope of this book to go into details about the different types of white blood cells. However, for the subsequent discussion of how vaccines work, we need to understand a little bit more about a few of these cells. Below, we'll take a look at both the white blood cells that are part of the native immune defense and those that participate in the adaptive immune response

The Neutrophils: First-Line Defenders

The most abundant white blood cells are the neutrophils, which play an important role in the innate immune defense. When they meet a microorganism, they react by secreting several substances, including a protein named HBP. The HBP protein attracts other white blood cells, such as monocytes, to the site of the infection and starts up the later phases of the immune response.

The B Lymphocytes and the T Lymphocytes

Other important cells are B lymphocytes and T lymphocytes. The B lymphocytes (B cells) are responsible for making highly specific antibodies against invading viruses and other microorganisms. Shortly after the B cells have met an antigen that they recognize, some of them start developing into plasma cells. Plasma cells are highly specialized cells whose function it is to make and secrete large amounts of antibodies to combat the invading virus.

The T lymphocytes (T cells) also play an important role in the immune defense. There exist several types of T cells; the more important are the T-helper cells and cytotoxic T cells. One of the major functions of the T-helper cells is to assist the B cells in creating a mature and strong antibody response against the invading viruses or other microorganisms. They also play an important role in transforming some of the B cells into memory cells.

The other important group of T cells, the T-cytotoxic cells, also have significant roles in the immune defense. Among other things, they secrete many compounds that assist in defeating the invading viruses. We'll examine the B and T cells in more detail below.

ADJUVANTS ENHANCE THE IMMUNE RESPONSE

An adjuvant is a compound that enhances the effectiveness of a vaccine. By using an adjuvant, the dose required to bring about an immune response may be reduced compared to the dose needed without an adjuvant. By using both a high vaccine dose and an adjuvant, a highly effective immune response may be generated.

Adjuvants mainly work by enhancing the native immune response that then intensifies the adaptive immune response. The simple compound alum hydroxide has been used for the decades as an adjuvant. Recently, newer and more effective adjuvants have been developed. We'll review some of the newer adjuvants when we look at the COVID-19 vaccine candidates in later chapters.

THE ADAPTIVE IMMUNE SYSTEM

The second part of our immune system is called the adaptive immune system. This name implies that it first starts working after we have met a microorganism for the first time. As the innate immune system, it mainly consists of white blood cells—but of types other than those involved in the innate immune system.

The two types of cells called B lymphocytes (B cells) and T lymphocytes (T cells), as mentioned above, play important roles in the adaptive immune defense. The "B" stands for bone marrow, whereas the "T" stands for thymus.

THE B CELLS AND T CELLS

Both B cells and T cells circulate in our blood and tissues, constantly monitoring for foreign entities. They carry specific receptors on their surface. Each B and T cell only carries receptors for one particular part of a microorganism. The part of the microorganism that reacts with the receptor on the B or T cell is called an antigen.

More precisely, the receptor on a B or T cell only binds to a tiny part of an antigen that's called an epitope. For simplicity, we'll generally use the term "antigen" in this book.

Our B cells may recognize more than 1,000 billion foreign antigens. Our T cells are even more capable, as they may recognize more than 100,000 billion foreign antigens. Both B and T cells have receptors on their surface that recognize a specific antigen. When they have recognized an antigen that matches their receptor, they start proliferating. They do not react to any other of the billions of antigens that they may meet. This makes the adaptive immune response highly specific.

As an example, a vaccine against the COVID-19 virus S protein only activates B and T cells that can recognize the S protein. The S protein contains many different antigens (epitopes). This means that many different B and T cells may react to the S protein. If the COVID-19 vaccine contains only the S protein, the B and T cells will not react to any other part of the COVID-19 virus. This makes the immune response highly specific.

If, in contrast, the vaccine consists of a whole inactivated COVID-19 virus, numerous B and T cells will react to the COVID-19 virus. They'll react not only to the S protein, but also to some of the other antigens on the surface of the COVID-19 virus. This results in a much broader immune response, but it will still be specific for the COVID-19 virus. However, some antibodies may react to COVID-19 antigens that are also found on other coronaviruses.

B CELLS AND THE ANTIBODY RESPONSE

When a B cell meets an antigen that it recognizes, for example the S protein on the COVID-19 virus, it starts proliferating. As a result of the proliferation, there will soon be many more B cells that recognize the COVID-19 S protein. The B cells start to secrete antibodies against the invading COVID-19 virus.

Initially, these antibodies are of the IgM type. The IgM antibodies are large antibody molecules that only bind weakly to the COVID-19 virus. A few days after the infection, the B cells start to secrete another type of antibody: the IgG antibody. IgG antibodies are more specific for the S protein than the IgM antibodies and bind strongly to the S protein. The production of IgG antibodies is highly important for the prevention or eradication of most viral infections.

Later in the course of the infection, some of the B cells start developing into plasma cells. Plasma cells are a highly specialized form of B cells, whose function it is to produce and secrete large amounts of antibodies that can neutralize the invading virus (here, the COVID-19 virus).

The antibodies secreted by the B cells and plasma cells are of fundamental importance in preventing or combating infections caused by viruses. Most effective vaccines against viruses work by generating a strong and long-lasting immune response that neutralizes the invading viruses and prevents them from causing disease.

NEUTRALIZING ANTIBODIES

To see if a vaccine candidate may be effective, the scientist takes blood specimens from the test animals or from the test subjects and measures the level of IgG antibodies or neutralizing antibodies.

Neutralizing antibodies are most often IgG antibodies, but the methods for measuring *just* IgG antibodies and neutralizing antibodies are different (see the gray box below).

IgG Antibodies and Neutralizing Antibodies

When scientists measure the level of IgG antibodies to the S protein, they add a small amount of serum (or plasma) from a blood specimen to a well in a plastic tray coated with the COVID-19 S protein. The IgG antibodies then

bind to the S protein and can be detected by adding a second antibody to the human IgG. The second antibody has been linked to an enzyme that can produce a colored compound.

This method only tells us if the specimen contains IgG antibodies. It does not say anything about whether or not the antibodies can neutralize the COVID-19 virus. One drawback of such a method is that it often also measures antibodies that only react weakly with the S protein. It is, however, useful for telling us if an antibody response has at all taken place in the vaccinated person.

The measurement of neutralizing antibodies is more complex. Here, the scientists first mix a small amount of the COVID-19 virus with the serum from a blood specimen from the vaccinated person. They usually use a modified COVID-19 virus, but for simplicity, here we'll just imagine that the measurement is made by adding the unmodified COVID-19 virus.

After some time, the mixture of the COVID-19 virus and serum is added to wells in another plastic tray coated with a cell line that the COVID-19 virus can infect. This may, for example, be Vero cells. (We'll learn more about Vero cells in Chapter 3.) If the Vero cells do not become infected, this tells us that there is no "free" COVID-19 virus present. The COVID-19 virus has thus been neutralized by the antibodies.

Neutralizing antibodies are, as their name indicates, capable of neutralizing the viruses. They bind so effectively to the virus or a part thereof, for example the S protein, that the virus cannot enter the human cells. Therefore, in the presence of the neutralizing antibodies, the virus cannot cause the disease.

Development of a high concentration of neutralizing antibodies in a vaccinated animal or test subject indicates that the vaccine will be effective. As we'll discuss in Chapter 4, the finding of a high concentration of neutralizing antibodies in small animals such as mice should not be given too much weight, whereas such observation in monkeys generally signifies that the vaccine also may be effective in humans.

NEUTRALIZING ANTIBODIES IN BLOOD FROM RECOVERED PATIENTS

People who've had a natural COVID-19 infection will most often have neutralizing antibodies to the COVID-19 virus in their blood. After the blood specimen has clotted, the neutralizing antibodies will be in the clear fluid above the clot: the serum. If the blood is prevented from clotting by adding an anticoagulant, the red blood cells will sediment and leave a clear fluid at the top. This is called plasma. Both the serum and plasma will contain neutralizing antibodies. In some newspaper articles, serum and plasma are used with the same meaning. Here, we'll use the term "serum."

Serum from people who have recovered from an infection is often called convalescence serum. Such serum may be used to treat patients who are very ill from a COVID-19 infection. This type of therapy has already been used successfully. It is called passive antibody therapy, because the patient's body does not have to make the antibodies. Passive antibody therapy has been used successfully for the earlier severe coronavirus infections: SARS and MERS.

The level of neutralizing antibodies in convalescent serum might also tell us something about how high the level of neutralizing antibodies after vaccination should be to offer protection against a COVID-19 infection. However, many different methods are being used to measure the level of neutralizing antibodies. In addition, only serum with high to very high levels (a titer above 160 or 320) of the COVID-19 neutralizing antibody is used for passive antibody therapy—to be on the safe side. It is therefore currently not possible to define precisely what the protective level of COVID-19 antibodies would be.

T-CELL RESPONSE TO VACCINATION

Besides the B cells, our immune system also consists of T cells. There are many different T-cell types. It is outside the scope of this book to give a description of each type and its role in immune defense. The neutralizing antibodies, produced by the B cells and plasma cells, seem to be the most important part of our immune defense against the COVID-19 virus. However, to work effectively, the B cells need assistance from the T cells.

There are two main types of T cells that here for simplicity are called the T4 cells and the T8 cells. The T4 cells are often called T-helper cells, whereas the T8 cells often are called cytotoxic cells—meaning that they can kill cells, including cells infected with viruses.

THE T4 CELLS ASSIST THE B CELLS

The T4 cells are needed to create an effective immune response against an invading virus. The T4 cells play an important role in assisting the B cells with maturing the antibody response, so that they make strong antibodies that can neutralize the virus. The T4 cells also assist the B cells with developing into memory B cells that remember the virus and quickly mount a strong antibody response, if they should ever meet the same virus again.

Both T4 cells and T8 cells may develop into memory T cells that may also be important for protection against the viral infection later.

The T cells secrete several compounds that play a fundamental role in the overall immune response. Among these are interferons and interleukins. (Don't be concerned about these names; here, we'll examine only one of them.) One of these interferons is Interferon γ (IFN γ). Both T4 and T8 cells secrete IFN γ, but IFN γ is mainly secreted by the former.

To determine if the T cells have been activated as a result of the vaccination, the scientists add a small amount of the vaccine to a blood specimen from the vaccinated subject. If this results in the release of IFN γ, it tells us that the vaccination has activated the T cells.

NATURAL IMMUNITY TO CORONAVIRUSES MAY LAST SOME MONTHS

As the COVID-19 virus has only been around for about six months, we don't know how long infected people will remain protected against a new infection.

After a natural infection with one of the common-cold coronaviruses, the antibodies seem to wane over the years. There are indications that natural immunity to the common-cold coronaviruses may last only a couple of years or even less. It has recently been proposed that immunity to the COVID-19 virus may only last between six and 12 months.

However, the good news is that vaccine schemes may be developed that may generate a much more effective and longer-lasting immune response than a natural infection with the COVID-19 virus.

THE STRENGTH AND DURATION OF THE IMMUNE RESPONSE

We don't know all the factors that determine the strength or duration of the immune response after a vaccination. We'll explore the more important factors below.

THE TYPE OF VACCINE ITSELF IS IMPORTANT

The type of vaccine is a highly important factor. Thus, live attenuated vaccines (Chapter 6) generally give a very strong antibody response after just a single vaccination. A booster dose is therefore not needed. As an example, one shot of a smallpox vaccine leads to lifelong protection. Today smallpox is eradicated.

Inactivated vaccines (Chapter 5) are often less effective in inducing an immune response. It may, therefore, be necessary to give the person two or even three doses to achieve a satisfactory protection against the virus. An adjuvant may also be needed to enhance the immune response. Four of the front-runners, which were in clinical trials as of June 24, were inactivated vaccines.

However, not all trials of inactivated COVID-19 vaccines include a booster dose or an adjuvant.

Non-replicating viral vector vaccines (Chapter 7) and subunit vaccines (Chapter 8) generally also give a weaker immune response than live attenuated vaccines. The immune response may be enhanced by the administration of two or three doses with an appropriate interval or by use of an adjuvant.

THE DOSE AND DOSING SCHEME ARE ALSO IMPORTANT

The dose of the vaccine is also important. It is, however, not so that more is always better. A high dose will usually, up to a certain threshold, give a stronger immune response—at least in the short term. Higher doses may be utilized to protect as many people as quickly as possible in an emergency.

However, a high dose may not necessarily lead to better B-cell memory. A more effective way to generate long-term B-cell memory and to enhance the antibody response, if the virus is met again, may be to give a low start dose and low booster dose(s) with long intervals (three to six months).

There may thus be a delicate balance between the wish to give a fast and strong primary antibody response and to prepare for an even faster and stronger secondary antibody response—should the COVID-19 virus ever be encountered again.

WILL THE COVID-19 VACCINE(S) PRODUCE A STRONG IMMUNE RESPONSE?

Among the 16 lead candidates in the COVID-19 vaccine race, there is no live attenuated vaccine or replicating viral vector vaccine. These two vaccine types generally give the strongest and longest-lasting immune response even after a single dose.

The other COVID-19 vaccine types currently (as of June 24) in the top-16 league are inactivated whole virus vaccines (four candidates), non-replicating viral vector vaccines (three candidates), subunit vaccines (three candidates), RNA vaccines (four candidates), and DNA vaccines (two candidates). These types of vaccines usually don't generate a strong and long-lasting immune response after a single shot. This makes it less likely, but not impossible, that only one dose would be enough to offer long-term protection. We'll look at each of the top 16 COVID-19 virus vaccine candidates and their likelihood of success in later chapters.

However, the goal for the current COVID-19 vaccines in development may not be to offer long-lasting protection. Their role would rather be to curtail or end the pandemic. Later, new vaccines or vaccine schedules—or even other types of vaccines—offering long-term protection may then be developed.

Furthermore, for several of the 16 COVID-19 vaccine candidates in clinical trials, vaccine schemes using more than one dose are being tested. In addition, in some trials, adjuvants are being used to further intensify the immune response. This gives us hope that it may be possible to develop an effective COVID-19 vaccine shortly—even though more than one shot may have to be given to ensure long-lasting protection.

ANTIBODY-DEPENDENT ENHANCEMENT

Antibodies following an infection or a vaccination do not always do a good job of protecting us from becoming ill—or from becoming ill again, if we already have been infected once. In some cases, antibodies may ease the entry of the virus into our cells and may hence *increase* instead of decreasing our risk of becoming ill.

It is not clear why antibodies sometimes may lead to the enhancement of an infectious disease. An antibody consists of two parts. One part binds to the antigen, for example the COVID-19 S protein, whereas the other part may bind to receptors on our immune cells. An IgG antibody is in the form of a "Y." The two arms bind to the antigen, whereas as the "leg" binds to our cell receptors.

One theory proposes that over time, the antibodies—particularly the non-neutralizing antibodies—become less able to bind to the antigen. They may still bind to the antigen, but they are no longer able to neutralize the antigen (the virus). Instead, they may enhance uptake of the antigen into some of our cells by binding to their antibody receptors.

Antibody-dependent enhancement has been observed for a number of viruses, including coronaviruses. It has been speculated that antibody-dependent enhancement may have played a role in patients infected with other coronaviruses before they got an infection with the COVID-19 virus. This has, however, not been proven.

In some of the ongoing clinical trials, the investigators plan to monitor for antibody-dependent enhancement. However, it should be recalled that it may take a long time before antibody-dependent enhancement develops—maybe a year or more. The antibody response first needs to weaken. In the rush to bring a COVID-19 vaccine to market as soon as possible, the observation time in the clinical trials may be too short to detect antibody-dependent enhancement. The same may apply to the animal testing performed prior to the clinical trials.

The best thing that the investigators can do is to monitor carefully for any indication of antibody-dependent enhancement and to perform various lab experiments for antibodies that could cause antibody-dependent enhancement.

My assessment is that there is a risk that antibody-dependent enhancement may occur for some of the COVID-19 vaccine candidates. How high the likelihood is, we don't know yet. However, from the clinical tests of SARS and MERS vaccines, the risk does not seem too high.

KEY TAKEAWAYS

Our immune system consists of the innate and adaptive immune system. Both play an important role in immunity after a vaccination.

The two more important cell types in the adaptive immune system are the B cells and the T cells. The B cells and the plasma cells make the antibodies that neutralize the COVID-19 virus. The generation of high levels of neutralizing antibodies after vaccination is the most important part of our immune response against the COVID-19 virus.

We don't know all the factors that determine the strength and duration of a vaccination. We do, however, know that some vaccine types (for example, live attenuated vaccines) are more effective than others (for example, inactivated vaccines).

The effectiveness of a vaccine may be intensified by several means. First, more than one dose may be given. Second, an adjuvant may be added to enhance the immune response. Third, the dose scheme may be optimized to give the best possible immune response. These means may be combined to mount a particularly effective immune response.

Although none of the top 16 COVID-19 vaccine candidates that are currently in clinical trials might be ideal, the option to develop a highly effective vaccination schedule gives us hope that one or more of the vaccine candidates may be sufficiently effective to curtail or end the COVID-19 pandemic ... when a sufficient number of doses becomes available.

REFERENCES

BC Centre for Disease Control. "Immunization Manual." accessed June 3. http://www.bccdc.ca/health-professionals/clinical-resources/communicable-disease-control-manual/immunization.

Bloch, E. M., S. Shoham, A. Casadevall, B. S. Sachais, B. Shaz, J. L. Winters, C. van Buskirk, B. J. Grossman, M. Joyner, J. P. Henderson, A. Pekosz, B. Lau, A. Wesolowski, L. Katz, H. Shan, P. G. Auwaerter, D. Thomas, D. J. Sullivan, N. Paneth, E. Gehrie, S. Spitalnik, E. A. Hod, L. Pollack, W. T. Nicholson, L. A. Pirofski, J. A. Bailey, and A. A. Tobian. 2020. "Deployment of convalescent plasma for the prevention and treatment of COVID-19." *J Clin Invest* 130 (6):2757-2765.

CDC. 2020. "Vaccine Effectiveness: How Well Do the Flu Vaccines Work?", Last Modified 2020, January 3, accessed June 3. https://www.cdc.gov/flu/vaccines-work/vaccineeffect.htm#:~:text=While%20vaccine%20effectiveness%20(VE)%20can, matched%20to%20the%20flu%20vaccine.

Lauritzen, B., J. Lykkesfeldt, R. Djurup, H. Flodgaard, and O. Svendsen. 2005. "Effects of heparin-binding protein (CAP37/azurocidin) in a porcine model of Actinobacillus pleuropneumoniae-induced pneumonia." *Pharmacol Res* 51 (6):509-14.

Li, L., and N. Petrovsky. 2016. "Molecular mechanisms for enhanced DNA vaccine immunogenicity." *Expert Rev Vaccines* 15 (3):313-29.

Muruato, AE et al. 2020. "A high-throughput neutralizing antibody assay for COVID-19 diagnosis and vaccine evaluation." bioRxiv, Last Modified May 22, 2020, accessed JUne 3. https://www.biorxiv.org/content/10.1101/2020.05.21.109546v1.

Salmons, B., P. Y. Lim, R. Djurup, and J. Cardosa. 2018. "Non-clinical safety assessment of repeated intramuscular administration of an EV-A71 VLP vaccine in rabbits." *Vaccine* 36 (45):6623-6630.

Schiller, J. T., and D. R. Lowy. 2015. "Raising expectations for subunit vaccine." *J Infect Dis* 211 (9):1373-5.

Schou, M., R. Djurup, K. Norris, and H. Flodgaard. 2011. "Identifying the functional part of heparin-binding protein (HBP) as a monocyte stimulator and the novel role of monocytes as HBP producers." *Innate Immun* 17 (1):60-9.

Sheridan, C. 2020. "Convalescent serum lines up as first-choice treatment for coronavirus." Last Modified May 7, accessed June 3. https://www.nature.com/articles/d41587-020-00011-1.

Siegrist, C-A. 2018. *Vaccine Immunology*. Edited by Plotkin SA. et al., *Plotkin's Vaccine*. Book.

Sztein, MB; Ahmed, R; and Crotty, S. 2017. *Recent Advances in Immunology That Impact Vaccine Development*. Edited by MM Levine, *New Generation Vaccines, 4th. Edition*: CRC Press.

Wan, Y., J. Shang, S. Sun, W. Tai, J. Chen, Q. Geng, L. He, Y. Chen, J. Wu, Z. Shi, Y. Zhou, L. Du, and F. Li. 2020. "Molecular Mechanism for Antibody-Dependent Enhancement of Coronavirus Entry." *J Virol* 94 (5).

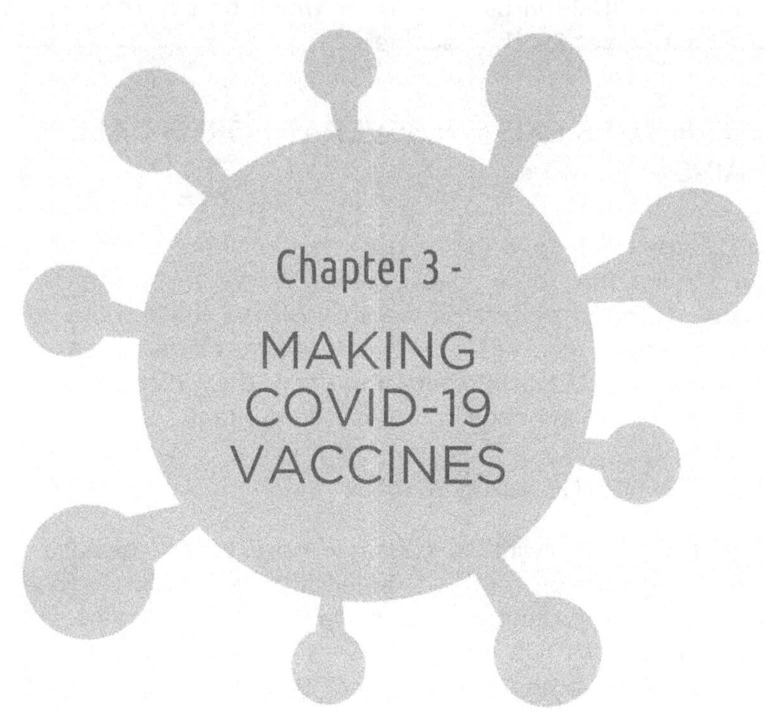
Chapter 3 -
MAKING
COVID-19
VACCINES

When researchers want to develop a new vaccine, the first thing they must do is to select a virus (or part of it) in order to make the vaccine. It's very important that the scientists choose the best possible target for the vaccine. Otherwise, the vaccine to be developed may be ineffective, may only protect some people, or may only partially protect the vaccinated subjects. So naturally, to make a vaccine against the COVID-19 virus, scientists must select a COVID-19 virus—or at least a part of it. The key question is: Which COVID-19 virus (strain), or which part of the virus, will be the best target for the vaccine?

MOST VIRUSES EXIST IN SEVERAL FORMS CALLED STRAINS

Most disease-causing viruses exist in many forms called "strains." Some strains frequently cause diseases, whereas others only infrequently infect people. Some strains may cause more severe disease courses, whereas others may cause milder diseases like the common cold. It's therefore important that scientists select a strain that frequently causes diseases in humans.

SELECTION OF THE VIRUS STRAIN

If one strain is thought to cause a more severe disease than others, it might be preferable to select that particular strain. As of this writing, it is not known with certainty if some strains cause a more severe COVID-19 disease course than others, but recently there has been some indication that this might actually be the case (see below).

It may be somewhat difficult to define what a virus strain is. Here, we may define it as a subtype of the COVID-19 virus that possesses some unique features that distinguish it from other subtypes of the COVID-19 virus. It might, for example, cause a milder or more severe disease course, or perhaps be more contagious.

SELECTION OF PART OF THE VIRUS AS A TARGET FOR THE VACCINE

If scientists want to make a vaccine against only a part of the COVID-19 virus, they must be very careful to select a part that is pivotal for the COVID-19 virus to cause the disease. For COVID-19 vaccines, this means that the subunit must contain spike proteins (S proteins) on the surface of the COVID-19 virus. You'll learn more about this later in the chapter.

THE COVID-19 VIRUS AND ITS STRAINS

Although the COVID-19 virus has only been around for about six months, it was recently found that it already exists in several strains.

THE COVID-19 VIRUS MUTATES QUITE OFTEN

Strains occur through mutation. As discussed in Chapter 1, the COVID-19 virus (like other RNA viruses) mutates often. However, far from all mutations lead to a new strain. In fact, most mutations do not differ much from their predecessor, and will cause the same type of disease as their predecessor if they should infect another person. Although such variants of the COVID-19 virus may have slightly different genes, they are not considered strains if no difference between them can be observed—regarding, for example, the severity of the disease or their ability to infect others.

WE ALREADY KNOW SEVERAL COVID-19 STRAINS

By the end of May 2020, more than five million people worldwide had been infected with COVID-19. In each of the infected subjects, the virus may have mutated. After some time, the many mutations created during the infection of millions of people may lead to new strains.

It is therefore unsurprising that several strains of the COVID-19 virus have already developed. The good news is that there is no sign that these strains differ much from each other, and the current prevailing opinion is that a vaccine developed against one COVID-19 strain will also be effective against all the other strains.

VACCINES AGAINST WHOLE VIRUSES

Some of the first and most successful vaccines that humans have developed—for example, the vaccines against smallpox, polio, and measles—have used whole viruses to produce the vaccine. As we'll learn in Chapters 5 and 6, whole viruses may be used to make inactivated vaccines (Chapter 5) or live attenuated vaccines (Chapter 6).

INACTIVATED VACCINES AGAINST THE WHOLE COVID-19 VIRUS

Developing an inactivated vaccine is often a relatively simple and fast task compared to developing a live attenuated vaccine or viral vector vaccine (Chapter 7). It is therefore unsurprising that four of the 16 front-runners (as of June 24) in the COVID-19 vaccine race are inactivated vaccines (Chapter 5).

As we'll see later in this chapter, the COVID-19 viruses grow easily in kidney cells from the African green monkey. These cells are called Vero cells. Vero cells are an established platform for the manufacturing of vaccines, so by using Vero cells, there is no need to design and develop a new cell line. In addition, ready-to-use manufacturing methods have been developed for the growth and purification of viruses in the Vero cells. Three of the inactivated vaccines against COVID-19 that are currently being tested in humans have been manufactured in Vero cells. We have no information about the manufacturing of the fourth inactivated vaccine. We'll examine the manufacturing of COVID-19 vaccine candidates in Vero cells later in this chapter.

VACCINES AGAINST ONLY PART OF THE COVID-19 VIRUS

To create an effective vaccine, one does not need to use the whole virus; it is possible to use only a part of the virus to make a vaccine.

VACCINES AGAINST THE COVID-19 SPIKE PROTEIN

COVID-19 is a virus in which the genes consist of RNA. It has both a capsid (as all viruses have) and an envelope. The envelope contains the spike proteins that are needed for the virus to enter human cells. The S proteins bind to a specific receptor on human cells (the ACE2 receptor). The part of the S protein that binds to the human ACE2 receptor is called the Receptor-Binding Domain (RBD).

The binding of the COVID-19 S protein to the ACE2 receptor makes it possible for the virus to enter the cells. This means that if the S proteins are blocked, for example by an antibody, it will not be possible for the virus to enter the human cells and infect the person.

A simple approach to making a vaccine against the COVID-19 virus would therefore seem to be to make the vaccine against the S proteins. In fact, there are several COVID-19 vaccine candidates in the pipeline that target the S protein. Several of the front-runners already in clinical trials thus target the S protein, though by use of different vaccine technologies (viral vector, RNA, DNA, or protein subunit vaccines). We'll review each of these approaches below and in later chapters.

VIRAL VECTOR VACCINES AGAINST THE COVID-19 S PROTEINS

To get the COVID-19 genes, which make the S proteins, into human cells, one needs to use a shuttle - also known as a viral vector. One of the most popular vectors for making vaccines is a virus that causes the common cold in many people, namely the adenovirus. Through genetic engineering, it's possible to build the wanted genes (in this case, the genes making the S proteins) from the COVID-19 virus into the adenovirus genes. The adenovirus will then carry the COVID-19 S protein genes into the human cells, and the body will mount an immune response against the S proteins.

However, the immune system may also make antibodies against the adenovirus genes, which may sometimes lead to a less effective immune response. We'll learn more about this problem and how to handle it in Chapter 7.

This is a popular way to develop vaccines, and as we'll see in Chapter 7, there are several COVID-19 vaccine candidates of this type in development. There is, however, no licensed vaccine based *solely* on an adenovirus vector on the market (Chapter 7)—despite the popularity of the technology, which has been in use for more than 30 years.

Vaccines based on viral vectors are usually not classified as subunit vaccines. Organizations like WHO place them in their own class: non-replicating viral vector vaccines. Nonetheless, some of the adenoviral vaccine candidates mentioned here express only the S proteins. The difference between adenovirus viral vector vaccines and the proper subunit vaccines is that the viral vector vaccines enter the human cells, where they start to produce the COVID-19 S proteins. In contrast, a proper subunit vaccine does not make any COVID-19 proteins inside our cells. They are made outside our body.

VACCINES AGAINST THE COVID-19 CAPSID OR PART THEREOF

It's also possible to make a COVID-19 vaccine against a part of the virus without having to use viral vector technology. A vaccine targeting the virus capsid or any part thereof is called a protein subunit vaccine. WHO distinguishes between vaccines targeting the whole capsid, called virus-like particles, and vaccines targeting a single capsid protein, called protein subunit vaccines.

In this book, I've included virus-like particle vaccines in the group of "protein subunit vaccines." When I finished editing the book (June 24), there was no virus-like particle COVID-19 vaccine in clinical trials, but there were three other protein subunit vaccines (see Chapter 8). The COVID-19 protein subunit vaccine candidates in clinical trials all target the S protein or a part thereof.

Protein subunit vaccines, whether virus-like particles or single-protein subunit vaccines, do not contain any genes. They therefore cannot cause the disease that they're intended to protect against. Protein subunit vaccines are very safe.

VACCINES USING THE COVID-19 RNA TO TRICK THE IMMUNE SYSTEM

As discussed in Chapter 1, a virus consists of a core in which the genes are located in the form of DNA or RNA. The genes are contained within a capsid. The capsid mainly or solely consists of proteins. Furthermore, some viruses, for example the COVID-19 virus, have a capsule around the capsid.

Today, it is technically possible to make a vaccine against only a part of the capsule, against a part of the capsid, or against the whole capsid. As we shall see later in Chapters 9 and 10, it is also possible to use the virus RNA or a DNA vector to create an immune response without having to vaccinate with the whole virus or any part of the capsid or capsule.

In this way, it may be possible to bypass the laborious work of making, purifying, and testing the whole virus. Instead, one may simply synthesize part of the COVID-19 virus RNA and inject it directly into people, so that the body believes it has been infected with the COVID-19 virus. As RNA is easy to synthesize and may be synthesized in large amounts within a short time, this approach has received a lot of attention, particularly in the news. We'll consider the RNA vaccine candidates in Chapter 9. Currently, no licensed vaccine based on the RNA technology exists, but several mRNA-based COVID-19 vaccines are already in clinical trials. Four of the 16 lead candidates in clinical trials are thus mRNA vaccines.

CELLS THAT CAN PRODUCE THE COVID-19 VIRUS VACCINES

Let's now briefly turn to the common approach to manufacturing virus vaccines in cells. The description of vaccine manufacturing below applies to inactivated vaccines, live attenuated vaccines, and viral vector vaccines, but not to all vaccine types. As an example, RNA vaccines are manufactured through chemical synthesis, which is a much simpler procedure.

It takes many, many viruses to make a vaccine. A single dose may contain millions or even billions of viruses. To be able to make a vaccine, we must therefore be able to grow the viruses to a considerable number.

In contrast to bacteria, which can grow in quite simple nutritious "soups" without any cells, any virus needs a cell to be able to replicate itself. Viruses are very simple organisms that cannot grow outside cells.

HOST CELLS

The cells used for growing viruses are called host cells. The host cell lines that are used for manufacturing viruses today are all continuous cell lines. In a cell line, all descendants are supposed to be identical to the original ancestor. The cells in a cell line therefore have the same properties.

Some important vaccines are still not manufactured in cell lines but in other cell types or in a similar substrate. Most flu vaccines are still grown in fertilized hens' eggs (called embryonated eggs in the industry). Other vaccines are made in chicken embryo fibroblasts (CEFs)—cells that are harvested from chicken embryos.

The cell lines used in vaccine manufacturing today are all immortal cell lines. Whereas a normal cell has a finite life span, immortal cells can, at least theoretically, live forever. Cells may become immortal through natural development or gene engineering.

Host cells are needed to manufacture inactivated vaccines (Chapter 5), live attenuated vaccines (Chapter 6), and viral vector vaccines (Chapter 7), as well as for some subunit and virus-like particle vaccines (Chapters 8 and 9). Host cells are not needed for, for example, RNA vaccines, which is one reason why there is currently so much interest in the development of an RNA vaccine. The manufacturing of the vaccine is much simpler and cheaper than the manufacturing of, for example, an inactivated vaccine.

NATURAL HOST CELLS

Viruses can obviously grow in certain tissues of the species, which they then infect. This means, for example, that the COVID-19 virus can grow in cells from humans—not necessarily in all cell types, but at least in cells from the airways. It is, however, not very practical to use such specialized cells. Among other things, it may take a long time to develop a cell culture of human airway cells.

Although viruses are often choosy about the cell type in which they will grow, they may grow in human immortal cell lines such as the PER.C6 cell line (see below) and in cell lines from monkeys, such as the Vero cell line (see below).

A CELL LINE FROM A HUMAN EMBRYO: THE PER.C6 CELL LINE

Viruses that can infect humans often grow in human cell lines. Such cell lines generally stem from an aborted embryo. An example of such a cell line is the PER.C6 cell line. The precursor of this cell line was isolated by a Dutch scientist back in 1985. It was then stored in liquid nitrogen until 1995, when scientists started to work on it to develop a cell line specifically for the manufacturing of pharmaceutical products.

In contrast to many other cell lines, the PER.C6 line was from the very beginning designed to make pharmaceutical products, including vaccines. In the late 90s, a pharmaceutical company called Crucell was founded based on this cell line. In the next few years, Crucell successfully developed several vaccine candidates and vaccines based on the PER.C6 cell line.

The PER.C6 cell line may be used to grow whole virus vaccines to be inactivated and live attenuated viruses. It may also be used to make subunit vaccines and adenovirus-based vector vaccines.

The PER.C6 cell line was immortalized by inserting a gene from the common cold adenovirus type 5. As we'll see in Chapter 6, adenovirus vector-based vaccines are missing a gene that's essential for replication—the E1 gene—and hence cannot replicate themselves. The PER.C6 line contains the E1 gene from adenoviruses and can therefore complement deficient adenoviruses with this gene. This means that many types of virus vector-based vaccines can grow in the PER.C6 line.

Whereas many whole viruses have been grown in the PER.C6 cell line and brought to the market, no adenovirus-based vaccine manufactured in the PER.C6 cell line has been approved for commercial use.

Crucell successfully established the PER.C6 cell line and the technology for making adenovirus-based vaccines as the PER.C6® and AdVac® platforms, which may be used to develop and manufacture almost any type of virus vaccines. In 2009, Crucell was taken over by Johnson & Johnson, which today owns the AdVac® and PER.C6® cell line technologies and platforms.

We'll examine the Johnson & Johnson COVID-19 vaccine candidate in more detail in Chapter 7.

THE HEK293 CELL LINE

The HEK293 cell was isolated from a human embryo. It is generally thought to be a kidney cell (hence the "K") but may have some characteristics of a nerve cell, too. In any case, it was modified by adenovirus to make it "immortal", and it contains the E1 genes that the non-replicating adenovirus viral vectors are missing. The non-replicating adenovirus vectors can therefore grow in HEK293 and other similar cell types. Due to the way the HEK293 cell line was constructed, there is a very small risk that it may exchange genes with an adenovirus vector. If, for example, the HEK293 gives back the E1 gene to the adenovirus vector, it would be able to replicate again, which may lead to unwanted immune response. The HEK293 cell is, however, a useful host cell platform and used for manufacturing of some of the COVID-19 vaccine candidates, for example, the ChAdOx1 vector vaccine from the Oxford group.

A CELL LINE FROM AN AFRICAN MONKEY: THE VERO CELL LINE

Back in 1962, Japanese scientists developed the Vero cell from a kidney cell from the African green monkey. The name comes from the language Esperanto; "Vero" is an abbreviation of "verda reno," which in Esperanto means green kidney.

The Vero Cell Line Is the Most Widely Used Cell Line for Vaccine Manufacturing

The Vero cell line is the most widely used cell line for the development of vaccines. Over the years, the cell line has been developed so that it can grow without being attached to any surface, whereas many other cell types need some surface to attach to in order to grow and replicate. (Such a surface may be provided by a simple plastic tray or by microbeads.) Vero cells don't need such a surface, and can therefore grow in a suspension culture, which makes it much easier, faster, and usually cheaper to scale up the manufacturing to large volumes. Today, it is possible to manufacture viruses in bioreactors of up to 10,000 liters or even more.

In addition, it can grow in media without the addition of sera from animals, which reduces the risk of the cell culture becoming contaminated with other viruses, other microorganisms, or prions (which may cause mad cow disease). These days most cell lines for the growth of viruses can grow without the addition of sera from animals, and it is today a requirement by regulatory authorities that animal sera is not used in any manufacturing step for a virus vaccine.

The Vero cell line has been used successfully for the manufacturing of a large number of viral vaccines and for the development and early manufacture of an even greater number of vaccine candidates.

The Vero Cell Is Well Known by Regulatory Authorities

The Vero cell is well known by regulatory authorities in the US, the EU, and elsewhere, and today it's considered a standard platform for the development and manufacture of virus vaccines. Vaccines manufactured in the Vero cell line are very safe.

For the development of new vaccines, particularly in emergency situations such as the current COVID-19 epidemic, the Vero cell line would be a suitable platform for the rapid development of a vaccine against the COVID-19 virus.

Vero cells may be used for the development and manufacturing of inactivated vaccines (Chapter 5) and live attenuated vaccines (Chapter 6).

MAKING BILLIONS OF VACCINE VIRUSES

When scientists have selected the virus or the virus antigen that will be the target for the vaccine, the first step is to make a master virus seed stock that can be used to create the vaccine. To simplify this description, let's use a virus to be inactivated as an example here.

THE VIRUS MASTER SEED STOCK

To make a master virus seed stock, we only need a small number of viruses. They are to be prepared under very carefully controlled conditions known as good manufacturing practice (GMP). The number of viruses needed is often produced in a small lab bottle containing 500 milliliters or 1,000 milliliters. This stock is then portioned out in small vials or ampoules, each containing (for example) 1 milliliter.

The ampoules are stored at a very low temperature in liquid nitrogen. Before they can be used, they need to undergo extensive and careful testing. The test is done to ensure that the master virus seed stock only contains the virus of interest—here, the COVID-19 virus. There should obviously be no other viruses, microorganisms, or substances that might harm humans in the master seed virus stock. The testing includes several tests for other viruses. It's outside the scope of this book to go into details regarding the testing of a virus seed stock. However, the testing process is quite lengthy and often lasts two to three months. The purpose is, as mentioned, to ensure that the vaccine made from the virus stock is very safe so that the vaccinated people aren't at risk of getting any disease after being vaccinated.

When scientists have a master virus seed stock, they could directly use it to make large amounts of COVID-19 viruses by infecting (or inoculating, as it's called) an appropriate host cell—for example, the Vero cell or the PER.C6 cell. However, by using this approach, the virus seed stock could be quickly used up. It is therefore customary not to use the master virus seed stock itself to manufacture the viruses.

Instead, scientists may first make a working virus seed stock. One vial of the master virus seed stock may then be used to make, for example, 500 vials of the working virus seed stock, which may again be used to manufacture several hundred lots of the COVID-19 virus vaccine. Using this approach, a master virus seed stock may last for many decades, and billions of doses can be made from the virus seed stock. Each dose will only contain viruses that are identical to the original master virus seed stock.

The working virus seed stock will have to undergo the same extensive testing as the master virus seed stock. This adds another two to three months to the timeline. In the current emergency situation, we may not have up to six months to test the virus seed stocks, and the scientists may decide to use the master virus seed stock to make the first few lots of the COVID-19 vaccine for the first studies in humans. This saves about three months.

The timeline for making the first COVID-19 vaccine lot for testing in animals could be significantly reduced by doing tasks in parallel. The master virus seed could, for example, be used to create the first lot while it is still being tested. This would be an unusual procedure but could likely be accepted if the manufactured vaccine lot is kept in quarantine until the master virus seed stock has been released for use by quality control and quality assurance.

MANUFACTURING THE FIRST LOT FOR THE FIRST CLINICAL TRIAL

For the first clinical trials in humans, scientists need only a small number of doses—often fewer than 1,000. However, some of the clinical trials of the COVID-19 vaccine candidates have planned to enroll several hundred or even several thousand patients. As each subject may need to be given two doses, the need for doses may easily go up to about 20,000 or more for some of the larger planned clinical trials. In addition, many doses (vials) are needed for lab testing and stability studies.

However, this number of doses is easily made in a small lab-scale bioreactor. Bioreactors come in many forms. A typical bioreactor, which is often used for the initial manufacturing of virus vaccines or recombinant proteins, is a bottle with a volume of about 15 liters, containing a stirrer to ensure that the host cells are appropriately mixed with the virus seed, and that the viruses and host cells are kept in suspension.

Besides the virus seed stock, scientists also need an appropriate host cell to grow the viruses. I've already discussed two of the most widely used host cell lines: the Vero cell and the PER.C6 cell. Both are established cell line platforms. This means that there already exist master cell banks and working cells banks of these host cell lines. In addition, methods to grow the viruses in these cells and to purify the vaccine already exist. This means that a new vaccine such as the COVID-19 vaccine can be made much faster than was possible just a few years back.

GROWING THE VACCINE VIRUSES

To make a virus vaccine, the scientists first need to grow the viruses to a very high number. This is often called the upstream process. Afterward, the scientists need to purify the vaccine viruses so that they do not contain any unwanted substances (other microorganisms, residuals from the host cells, etc.).

To make the first lot in a small bioreactor, the scientists first have to grow the host cells to a very large number. This is simply done by adding a working cell bank ampoule to the bioreactor and some growth medium. Such growth media are today off-the-shelf products that are easily available. It normally takes three to four days, sometimes up to a week, to get a sufficient number of host cells. When the bioreactor is filled with an appropriate number of host cells, the next step is simply to add the virus seed stock to the cells. In this way, the host cells become infected with the virus. Adding the viruses to a host cell is called inoculation.

After the inoculation, the viruses will infect the cells and start to replicate inside them. Usually, one only adds one virus per 10 or

100 host cells. Such a small number of viruses obviously cannot infect all the host cells directly. However, as the viruses can replicate inside the cells, the descendants of the original virus seeds can infect many more host cells. Therefore, after a few days, all host cells will be infected. The number of host cells in a 10-liter bioreactor is very large—often 100 billion cells or more. Each cell may contain many viruses, often 100 or more, so a 10-liter bioreactor may altogether contain more than 100,000 billion viruses.

When the number of virus peaks, it is time to harvest the viruses. Some viruses spontaneously leave the host cells, whereas others may remain inside the host cell. To obtain the best possible virus yield, it may be needed to get the viruses out of the host cells when they are harvested. This can be done through various simple means, for example freezing and thawing the virus harvest. Freezing and thawing break up the host cell membranes and release the vaccine viruses inside the host cells. Alternatively, one may use ultrasound. The sound waves at very high frequencies (inaudible to the human ear) break up the host cell membranes and release the vaccine viruses.

PURIFYING THE VIRUSES

Before the viruses may be used to make a vaccine, they need to be purified. After the harvest, the viruses are found in a "soup," in which there are also host cells, growth medium, and possibly other unwanted components such as any chemicals used during the manufacturing of the viruses.

All these unwanted compounds need to be fully removed before the viruses can be used as a vaccine. This can be done with relatively simple technologies, where the components in the soup are sorted after their electric charge or their size. It is outside the scope of this book to go into details of the purification processes; however, it should be noted that for the most-often-used platforms—the Vero cell platform and the PER.C6 platform—such purification methods have been well established and have shown their value for manufacturing numerous vaccine candidates and licensed vaccines. There is therefore no need for any new invention or development here. In addition, vaccines made by these standard technologies have been proven to be very safe, as they have been given to millions of people.

The existence of a standard purification technology saves a lot of time and clearly simplifies the task of making a new COVID-19 vaccine. The purification of, for example, a 10-liter virus harvest often takes only a few days. This means that a small lot of a COVID-19 vaccine may be made in a couple of weeks.

TESTING THE VIRUS BULK

When the virus vaccine bulk has been manufactured, it must undergo numerous stringent tests to ensure that it does not contain any unwanted microorganisms (bacteria, other viruses, etc.) or residuals from the host cells (for example, host cell DNA). The test panel is very comprehensive and may take two to three months.

Some of the tests are highly specialized and only available from a limited number of contract research organizations. The major players in the vaccine business probably have their own test facility where they can carry out all the needed tests.

When all test results are available, they will need to be reviewed by first the company's quality control and then its quality assurance departments. Although this seems to be a simple task, aberrant results do occur, and it may take some time to evaluate the importance of any such aberrant finding. In a worst-case scenario, a test may have to be repeated.

TIMELINE FOR MAKING THE VACCINE

Altogether, it should be possible to make the first bulk lot of a COVID-19 vaccine within three to four months, when the cell bank and virus seed stock are available.

MAKING THE VACCINE READY FOR USE

We have seen above how a vaccine may be manufactured. The outcome of these processes is often called the bulk vaccine or the vaccine substance. Before we can administer it to an animal or a human, it must be filled into a vial, syringe, nasal spray, or another suitable container that is easy to use.

FILLING THE VACCINE INTO VIALS OR SYRINGES

There are many ways to administer a vaccine. Most often, the vaccine is given as an injection under the skin or into a muscle. A vaccine may, however, also be given as a nasal spray, put on a piece of sugar to be taken by the mouth, or even injected by use of a "gene gun" (Chapter 10).

All 16 COVID-19 vaccines that are currently (June 24) being tested on humans are administered as an injection. The preferred way of administration is to give the vaccine as an injection into a muscle. This means that the vaccine substance must be filled into vials or syringes before it can be given to any test animal or subject.

For the animal studies that precede the clinical trials and for the clinical trials themselves, it is generally an easy task to manufacture a sufficient number of vials or syringes. The vaccine must obviously be sterile, so the filling into vials or syringes must take place under carefully controlled conditions. This can be done in most labs and small manufacturing units.

FILLING ONE BILLION DOSES OF A COVID-19 VACCINE

Ordering a few thousand vials or syringes is generally no problem. However, some institutions and companies have stated that they can deliver up to or more than one billion doses of COVID-19 vaccines within this year or early next year. This is quite a different task.

In my experience from working in big pharma, no supplier stockpiles such large amounts. For example, just to get 100 million glass vials delivered within a short time may be a huge challenge, if at all possible. The same applies to syringes and needles.

The now former director of the US Biomedical Advanced Research and Development Authority (BARDA), Rick Bright, shares this opinion. March 12, he notified HHS officials that all major pharmaceutical tubing suppliers are sold out of borosilicate tubing, which are used to manufacture the glass vials. Bright also estimated that between 650 million to 850 million needles and syringes would be needed just for the US market, and that it might take up to two years to make that quantity.

Even if it were possible to purchase such quantities of vials, syringes, and needles, the chances that any big pharma or contract manufacturer has a spare filing capacity of this size are, in my experience, very low.

The major pharma players participating in the COVID-19 vaccine race should be aware of this logistical challenge, but such large-scale manufacturing usually takes more than just a month or a few months to plan and implement.

However, in this context, it may be worth noting that in 2015, the global capacity for making a flu vaccine was about seven billion doses per year. This would mean that if the entire flu vaccine manufacturing capacity could be made available to manufacture COVID-19 vaccines, it might be doable to make billions of doses within a year.

The manufacturing of flu vaccine bulk generally uses manufacturing technologies, which are not suitable for making a COVID-19 vaccine. However, the equipment used for filling the flu vaccines into vials or syringes could be used for COVID-19 vaccines. This would obviously reduce the capacity for the filling of flu vaccines, so decision makers would have to decide which vaccine to prioritize.

Another solution would be to design and construct new filling factories. The regulatory authorities have very stringent requirements for such large-scale filling units, which therefore need to be tested and qualified before they can be used. This may take considerable time. Building and testing a new filling facility often takes a couple of years.

The availability of materials (vials, syringes, and needles) and the capacity for filling the vaccine into vials may hence become a bottleneck for any large-scale manufacturing of a COVID-19 vaccine. For each of the front-runner projects, we will in subsequent chapters assess whether the timeline for manufacturing the vaccine and filling of the vaccine appears to be realistic.

KEY TAKEAWAYS

Recent developments in vaccine manufacturing technologies have greatly reduced the time for the development and manufacturing of new vaccines.

The use of continuous cell lines such as the Vero cell line or the PER.C6 cell line makes it possible to manufacture the first lot for testing in animals and clinical trials in less than three months once the COVID-19 virus seed has been made.

Conducting tasks in parallel may significantly reduce the timeline for making the first COVID-19 vaccine lot. The testing of the virus seed may, for example, be done in conjunction with the use of the seed for manufacturing the first lot.

Usually, there would be no bottleneck for manufacturing small amounts of the COVID-19 vaccines or for filling the vaccine into vials or syringes.

Delivering one billion vaccines before the end of 2020 or by early 2021 would likely be a big challenge. Whereas some technologies might be able to deliver the needed vaccine in bulk within this time frame, filling vials with the vaccine might become a bottleneck.

REFERENCES

Alphagreen Team. 2020. "COVID-19: vaccine research & development." Last Modified April 29, accessed May 22.

Barrett, P. N., W. Mundt, O. Kistner, and M. K. Howard. 2009. "Vero cell platform in vaccine production: moving towards cell culture-based viral vaccines." *Expert Rev Vaccines* 8 (5):607-18.

Gleen, G. 2020. "NVX-CoV2373 Vaccine for COVID-19." Last Modified May 13, accessed May 23. https://novavax.com/download/files/2020-05-13WVCWebinarCOVID19v3.pdf.

Healthline. 2020. "COVID-19 Will Mutate — What That Means for a Vaccine." accessed May 22. https://www.healthline.com/health-news/what-to-know-about-mutation-and-covid-19.

Johnson & Johnson. 2020. "Johnson & Johnson Announces a Lead Vaccine Candidate for COVID-19; Landmark New Partnership with U.S. Department of Health & Human Services; and Commitment to Supply One Billion Vaccines Worldwide for Emergency Pandemic Use." Last Modified March 30, accessed May 24. https://www.jnj.com/johnson-johnson-announces-a-lead-vaccine-candidate-for-covid-19-landmark-new-partnership-with-u-s-department-of-health-human-services-and-commitment-to-supply-one-billion-vaccines-worldwide-for-emergency-pandemic-use.

Kirschweger, G. 2003. "Crucell: biopharmaceuticals--as human as they get." *Mol Ther* 7 (1):5-6.

Korber B, Fischer WM, Gnanakaran S et al. 2020. "Spike mutation pipeline reveals the emergence of a more transmissible form of SARS-CoV-2." BioRxiv, Last Modified May 5, accessed 3 July. https://www.biorxiv.org/content/10.1101/2020.04.29.069054v2.

Novavax. 2020. "Evaluation of the Safety and Immunogenicity of a SARS-CoV-2 rS (COVID-19) Nanoparticle Vaccine With/Without Matrix-M Adjuvant." Last Modified May 15, accessed May 23. https://clinicaltrials.gov/ct2/show/NCT04368988?term=vaccine&recrs=a&cond=covid-19&draw=2&rank=10.

Ooij, M van. 2017. "Use of platform technologies for Adenovirus-vectored vaccines." accessed May 25. https://www.ema.europa.eu/en/documents/presentation/presentation-case-study-3-use-platform-technologies-adenovirus-vectored-vaccines-session-2-mark-van_en.pdf.

Paillet, C., G. Forno, R. Kratje, and M. Etcheverrigaray. 2009. "Suspension-Vero cell cultures as a platform for viral vaccine production." *Vaccine* 27 (46):6464-7.

Serebrov, M. 2020. "Shortage of needles, syringes looms in race to develop COVID-19 vaccine." Bioworld, Last Modified May 8, accessed June.

https://www.bioworld.com/articles/434969-shortage-of-needles-syringes-looms-in-race-to-develop-covid-19-vaccine.

Shen, C. F., C. Guilbault, X. Li, S. M. Elahi, S. Ansorge, A. Kamen, and R. Gilbert. 2019. "Development of suspension adapted Vero cell culture process technology for production of viral vaccines." *Vaccine* 37 (47):6996-7002.

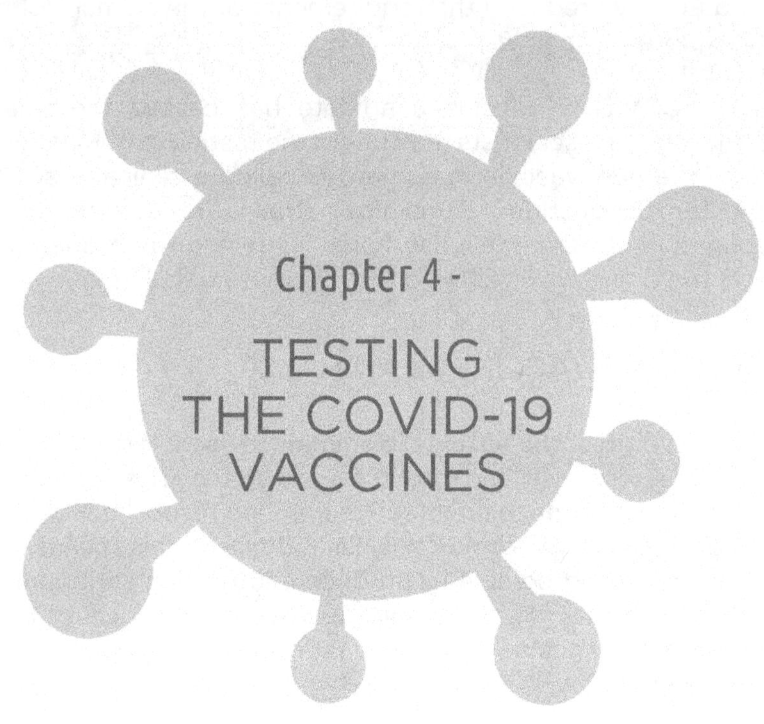
Chapter 4 -

TESTING
THE COVID-19
VACCINES

Before any vaccine is given to the first human, it is usually first tested in animals. First, the scientists test whether the vaccine is effective in animals. It should as a minimum generate neutralizing antibodies against COVID-19, and it should preferably also protect against the COVID-19 disease. Second, the scientists assess whether the vaccine causes any harm to the animals. The testing in animals often takes a long time. To speed up the development of COVID-19 vaccines, regulatory authorities in the US and EU have reduced the requirements of the animal testing. We'll explore this below.

When a COVID-19 vaccine candidate has passed the animal testing stage, the scientists may begin the testing in humans. The testing of a new vaccine in humans is called a clinical trial. The scientists conducting a clinical trial are often called investigators—a term we'll use here. There are three phases of clinical trials, and we'll examine them in more detail below.

TESTING THE VACCINE IN ANIMALS

Scientists first test the vaccine in animals to see if it can produce an immune response and protect against the disease. A new vaccine should produce an effective immune response. For most vaccines, including vaccines against COVID-19, this means that the vaccine should be able to produce neutralizing antibodies in the animals. It may be an advantage if it also produces a T cell response. If the vaccine generates antibodies or T cells, it is said to be immunogenic.

In traditional vaccine development, scientists often also test whether the vaccine can protect against the disease that it targets. This is often more difficult than testing whether the vaccine is immunogenic, because most species do not get the same disease(s) as humans. However, for the COVID-19 disease, rhesus monkeys are often used to test whether a COVID-19 vaccine candidate is effective (see further details below). This is usually done through a challenge test, by which the animals are exposed to the COVID-19 virus after they have been vaccinated. If they don't become ill, or seriously ill, the vaccine is able to protect against the disease. It is said to be effective.

Some scientists prefer to distinguish between efficacy and effectiveness. Efficacy may be defined as the performance under ideal and controlled circumstances, whereas effectiveness refers to the performance under "real-world" conditions. Even though clinical trials are meticulously planned and carried out, they do take place in the real world. Deviations from the plan occur, and unexpected incidents happen. I therefore prefer the term "effectiveness," which we'll use in this book.

When a vaccine candidate has been shown to be effective (immunogenic and/or protective), the scientists will then test to evaluate whether it is also safe.

They assess whether the vaccine causes adverse events or damage to the organs in the animals. If this is not the case, the vaccine is regarded as sufficiently safe to be tested in the first few humans.

Below, we'll explore the animal effectiveness tests in more detail. We'll also look at how scientists and vaccine companies—in collaboration with regulatory authorities (the FDA in the US and the EMA in the EU)—may cut some corners to speed up the development of a COVID-19 vaccine.

DOES THE VACCINE PROTECT AGAINST COVID-19?

Scientists typically start by testing the effectiveness of the vaccine in small animals such as mice and rats. However, unless some genetic engineering has been done to the animals, mice and rats don't usually get the same illness as humans when infected with COVID-19. It is possible to make an "animal model" for a human disease in mice and rats through genetic engineering, but this is a lengthy process.

Testing the vaccine in these small animals is still useful. When injected with the vaccine, a mouse will, as a human, start making antibodies and specific T cells against the vaccine (see Chapter 2). Scientists often use mice to see whether the vaccine can produce an antibody response in the animals—and in particular to see whether it can make neutralizing antibodies. This is the first step in showing that the vaccine is effective.

Often, the level of antibodies produced in mice is very impressive. However, one cannot predict whether the vaccine will produce the same level of neutralizing antibodies in humans. On the other hand, if a vaccine is not capable of creating a high level of neutralizing antibodies in mice, it is questionable whether it would be effective in humans.

TESTING THE COVID-19 VACCINE IN MICE

Several COVID-19 vaccine candidates have already been tested extensively in mice. Scientists have studied the generation of IgG antibodies, neutralizing antibodies, and T cells as responses to the vaccination.

Mice Differ From Humans

When interpreting the results, it should be remembered that mice are very different from humans; this includes their immune system. The limitations of using mice as model organisms for human infections have been repeatedly stressed in scientific papers. Many other vaccine candidates that have shown promising results in mice failed to be effective in humans. Although these limitations are well known, they are only briefly mentioned in some of the published studies of COVID-19 vaccine candidates in mice.

How Do We Know Whether a Vaccine Is Effective?

To consider a COVID-19 vaccine effective, scientists generally require that the vaccine creates neutralizing antibodies (see Chapter 2). The strength of the antibody response is often measured as how many times the blood (serum) can be diluted before the test becomes negative. This is called the titer. If a serum can be diluted 160 times, before the antibody can no longer be detected, the titer is expressed as 1:160 or 160. Here we'll use the latter way of expressing the titer.

The titer of antibodies in mice vaccinated with the COVID-19 vaccines is often impressive, with the IgG antibody response reaching titers of 4,000 or more, and with the titer of neutralizing antibodies reaching 1,000 or more.

Some scientists claim that the titers found in mice are much higher than the titers found in the blood (serum) of patients who had recovered successfully from a COVID-19 infection. Such serum is called convalescence serum. They see this as evidence that the vaccine will then also be effective in humans, but as mentioned, this is not always the case. There's an old saying in vaccine development (attributed to Dr. David B. Weiner, University of Pennsylvania, USA): "Mice lie, and monkeys exaggerate." This simply means that animal experiments are not always predictive of how the vaccine will work in humans.

TESTING COVID-19 VACCINES IN RHESUS MONKEYS

Rhesus macaques, here called rhesus monkeys, are Old World monkeys that approximately 25 million years ago separated as species from humans. Rhesus monkeys are much more similar to humans than mice, including their immune response to a vaccination.

The rhesus monkey has been the preferred model for the study of several human diseases, including many infectious diseases. It is often assumed that the results obtained in rhesus monkeys can be used to predict what will happen when humans are vaccinated. While this is the case in many situations, it is not always so.

Rhesus monkeys can be used to assess whether a COVID-19 vaccine is able to produce neutralizing antibodies, and whether it can protect against the COVID-19 disease. This can be done in the same experiment.

Does the Vaccine Produce Neutralizing Antibodies?

The monkeys are first vaccinated with the COVID-19 vaccine. The scientists may use the same dose as intended for the vaccination of humans, or they may use a slightly lower dose. At suitable intervals after the vaccination, the level of neutralizing antibodies in blood specimens is measured. If neutralizing antibodies are produced as a result of the vaccination, the COVID-19 vaccine is immunogenic.

Does the Vaccine Protect Against the COVID-19 Disease?

Shortly after the last dose has been given, the monkeys may be infected with the COVID-19 virus. This can be done by administering a COVID-19 virus specimen into their nose, throat, or windpipe. If the monkeys do not become ill or only get a mild COVID-19 disease, the COVID-19 vaccine candidate is protective.

Can Monkey Experiments Predict Effectiveness in Humans?

In some of the ongoing clinical trials, the company testing the vaccine in humans has announced that their vaccine candidate has been shown to produce neutralizing antibodies in humans. However, to date (June 24), no results of the 16 ongoing clinical trials have been published in the clinical trial registers or in any scientific publication.

To my knowledge, there has not yet been any formal comparison of the level of neutralizing antibodies found in animal experiments with those observed in humans. We therefore do not know whether the level of neutralizing antibodies seen in monkeys may predict the levels to be found in humans.

Only one of the currently (June 24) ongoing 16 clinical trials is attempting to assess whether the COVID-19 vaccine candidate can actually protect against the COVID-19 disease. The results of this trial conducted by the Oxford group (see Chapter 7) have not been reported yet. We hence do not yet know whether the neutralizing antibody level will predict the ability of the vaccine to protect against COVID-19 disease.

IS THE VACCINE SAFE IN ANIMALS?

Before any vaccine can be tested in humans, it must usually undergo a stringent evaluation in animals through a toxicology study (often just called a tox study). A tox study differs in several ways from animal effectiveness studies, which we have reviewed above.

First, the goal is to demonstrate that the vaccine is safe. It should not cause any harm to organs, and it should not cause serious inflammation or pain at the injection site. Second, the requirements of a tox study are much more formal than those of an effectiveness study. These requirements differ from country to country. It is outside the scope of this book to go into any details about this.

SELECTING THE VACCINE

The first challenge in doing a tox study is to have the right material: the right vaccine lot. Regulatory authorities prefer that the same lot is used for tox studies and the subsequent clinical trial. This is not always possible due to time limitations or scarcity of materials. The tox studies may therefore have to be done with a lot other than the one used in the clinical trial. The scientists must then document that the two lots are identical regarding all important parameters.

SELECTING THE ANIMAL SPECIES

The next challenge for a tox study is to select a relevant animal species. There is no requirement that the animal species selected for the tox studies should be able to get the same disease or a similar disease as humans get from the viral infection. In practice, mice, rats, or rabbits are often used in tox studies of vaccines. For vaccines, it is usually sufficient to use only one animal species.

The purpose of a tox study is to see whether the vaccine causes any harm to the test animal. To have a reasonable margin of safety, the test animals are often given much higher doses per kilogram of body weight than humans.

SELECTING THE NUMBER OF DOSES

Even though the scientists may want to give the human test subjects only one shot of the vaccine, regulatory authorities expect that the animals in the tox study will be given at least two doses—that is, one dose more than is intended for humans. Therefore, if the scientists plan to give a prime dose and a booster dose (two doses in total), the tox study should include three doses.

SELECTING THE TIME BETWEEN DOSES

If more than one dose of the vaccine is given to humans, there is often a long period between the first dose (prime dose) and the second dose (boost dose). That period is at least several weeks but may be up to several months. Such a long time between each dose is rarely possible in a tox study, where the dose interval is often squeezed down to only two or three weeks.

In a tox study, the animals need to be observed for some time after the last dose to exclude the possibility that toxic side effects may occur later in the course. A tox study may therefore easily last several months. It also takes the pathologist time to examine the animals and write the report. A realistic time frame for a tox study with three doses would be no less than 12 weeks. This obviously would put a limit on how fast a new vaccine can be developed if the standard protocol is followed. The tox study report is a highly important part of any application for starting a clinical trial in human subjects.

CUTTING CORNERS IN ANIMAL STUDIES

Already in March 2020, regulators in the US (the FDA) and EU (the EMA) held a joint meeting to discuss the animal experiment data needed to start testing the COVID-19 vaccine candidates in humans. They agreed that the data usually requested to start testing in humans might not be needed for all vaccine candidates.

Among other things, scientists do not need to provide data for the effectiveness of the vaccine prior to starting the first test in humans. In addition, the tox data normally requested to start a Phase 1 trial (see below) may not be needed for all vaccine candidates. If tox data exist from similar vaccines manufactured through the same platform technology, they may be used instead.

Regulatory authorities' willingness to cut some corners in the tox studies allows things to happen much faster than usual. As an example, the US company Moderna (see Chapter 9) started clinical trials with their RNA vaccine just 10 weeks after the COVID-19 gene sequence from the original Wuhan strain was published. This would not have left enough time for a standard tox study.

I don't know how Moderna achieved such fast progress. They might have conducted a very basic tox study. It doesn't need to take more than six to eight weeks to get the basic tox data for a two- to three-dose study with 14 days between each dose.

Another possibility is that Moderna based the assessment of toxicity of their COVID-19 RNA vaccine on studies of other RNA vaccines. Moderna had already manufactured several other RNA vaccine candidates and tested them in humans prior to the COVID-19 disease outbreak.

TESTING THE STABILITY OF THE VACCINE

Before a vaccine may be used in humans, it should also be shown that it would be stable for the planned time of the human trial. It is therefore common practice to start the stability studies at the same time as the tox studies. This way, it is possible to have at least three months' stability data when applying for starting the clinical trial.

CUTTING CORNERS IN STABILITY STUDIES

As with the tox studies, it is also possible to cut corners for the stability studies. It is desirable, but not always needed, to have shown that the vaccine is stable for at least three months before testing it on humans. The main reason for this is that no scientist or company usually wants to take the risk that the vaccine will become inactive during the test in humans.

An alternative is to start human testing based on only one month's stability and continue to follow the stability while the testing is running. Should it turn out that the vaccine becomes ineffective after, for example, two months, the study in humans can then be interrupted at that time.

TESTING IN HUMANS: CLINICAL TRIALS

When the animal studies and the tox studies have been completed and reported, the scientist can apply for permission to start testing the vaccine candidate in humans. The testing of a new vaccine candidate (or another drug) in humans is called a clinical trial. The scientist conducting the clinical trial is called an investigator. The lead investigator is the study director. The organization, company, or person overseeing and usually also financing the clinical trial is called the sponsor.

OPEN AND BLINDED CLINICAL TRIALS

To ensure that any effect of a vaccine is due to the vaccine itself, the clinical trial often includes various controls. Such controls may be another vaccine, the adjuvant alone (if an adjuvant is used with the COVID-19 vaccine), or simply saline. The COVID-19 vaccine is often called the active compound. A control is often called a placebo. If used in blinded trials (see below), the placebo must look exactly like the active vaccine.

A clinical trial may be designed as an open or blinded trial. In an open trial, the doctors, nurses, lab technicians, and participants all know which type of vaccine (active or placebo) and dose each participant receives. Open trials are primarily used in the early phases of the vaccine testing in healthy volunteers, particularly in Phase 1 trials.

In a blinded trial, none of the people involved in the study—doctors, nurses, technicians, or test subjects—knows which compound a participant receives. The label on the vial or syringe with the vaccine or control does not reveal what the compound is. This information is saved in a code, which is first opened when the trial has been completed.

REQUIREMENTS FOR CLINICAL TRIALS

The most important requirement for a clinical trial is that there should be a reasonable balance between the benefit and risk for the trial participants. For a vaccine against an infectious disease, the safety requirements need to be very high. After all, the people who will eventually be vaccinated are healthy and may not catch the infection at all.

In contrast, people suffering from a disease such as hypertension may benefit from a drug against hypertension. For patients suffering from cancer, a new drug may be their only hope. In clinical trials of such drugs, a greater risk may be taken because there may be a substantial benefit.

Please note that this does not mean that there is no benefit of vaccinating people once a COVID-19 vaccine becomes available. If, for example, 10% of the population each year get the COVID-19 infection, there would be a substantial benefit of vaccinating people. The more people who become infected, the higher the benefit is. If many of the infected people become severely ill or die, the benefit of vaccination with a COVID-19 vaccine will obviously also increase.

The Requirements Vary From Country to Country

The requirements for an application for testing new drug candidates in humans vary from country to country. In the US and the EU, the requirements are quite similar, although the formats in which the applications need to be presented are somewhat different. Other countries may follow the US rules (FDA rules) or the EU rules (EMA rules), or they may have their own.

In some countries, the requirements may be more stringent or less stringent than the requirements in the US or the EU. It is therefore important that the sponsor who's responsible for the clinical trials decides right from the start where they want the clinical trial to take place. Early contact with local authorities often saves much trouble later.

Deciding on the country for the clinical trial early on in vaccine development also has the advantage that the demanding paperwork can be initiated before the results from the clinical trial become available.

In the US, an application to start a clinical trial is called an Investigational New Drug Application (IND). In the EU, it's called a Clinical Trial Application (CTA).

When regulatory authorities receive such an application, they obviously need some time to review it to ensure that the vaccine candidate is safe for use in the first humans. The review process usually takes several months.

CUTTING CORNERS WHEN APPLYING TO START A CLINICAL TRIAL

As mentioned above, it saves a lot of time when the sponsor of a clinical trial contacts the regulatory authority early in the process. This way, the requirements of the study can be discussed early and any dispute resolved.

The protocol for the clinical trial and the other paperwork needed to start a clinical trial can be initiated long before the recruitment of participants begins.

Lastly, regulatory authorities offer "fast-track" schemes, where the time requested for review is reduced compared to the standard protocol.

THE THREE PHASES OF CLINICAL TRIALS

Any new vaccine candidate must go through three phases of clinical trials in humans: Phase 1, Phase 2, and Phase 3.

The Usual Approach: One Phase at a Time

The usual approach is to complete one phase before the next is initiated—and to have a break before the next phase. This means, for example, that Phase 2 will not begin before Phase 1 is completed.

There are several reasons for conducting the clinical trials this way. First, this approach exposes the least possible number of humans to any harm that the vaccine could cause. Second, it saves money when the next phase is not initiated until the preceding phase has been properly assessed. For example, should it turn out that the vaccine is unsafe in a Phase 1 trial, there would be no thought of continuing the clinical trials. (Doing so would also be ethically questionable.) Third, it may give the scientists time to modify the vaccine or the vaccine schedule, if needed.

The Pandemic Approach: Overlapping Between Phases

To speed up the clinical trial process, it is inevitable that more risks will have to be taken (both financial- and safety-related risks). However, it's possible to accelerate the clinical trial course and reduce the time between the three phases in a way that minimizes any additional risk(s) to the study participants.

One way to speed up the clinical trial is to let the subsequent phase overlap with the preceding phase. The sponsor may, for example, apply for a combined Phase 1/2 trial. However, the sponsor will only progress to testing the vaccine in a larger group of humans (Phase 2) when the safety of the vaccine has been found satisfactory in a smaller group of healthy humans (Phase 1). By using the same application to the authorities, a lot of time can be saved. In addition, recruitment for the next phase can be initiated early in the course—already before Phase 1 is completed.

THE SCOPE OF EACH PHASE OF THE CLINICAL TRIAL

As mentioned above, there are three different phases of clinical trials: Phase 1, Phase 2, and Phase 3.

THE PHASE 1 TRIAL

The purpose of a Phase 1 trial is primarily to ensure that the vaccine is safe. There is no requirement or need to demonstrate that the vaccine is also effective in this phase. However, to save time—especially in a situation as urgent as the COVID-19 pandemic—most scientists would prefer to also include some measures for effectiveness in the Phase 1 trial.

The easiest way to test for effectiveness is to take blood specimens at appropriate time intervals from the vaccinated people and to examine the specimens for any occurrence of various types of antibodies, such as IgG antibodies and neutralizing antibodies. This is being done in all ongoing clinical studies of COVID-19 vaccines. The production of neutralizing antibodies in the vaccinated subjects shows that the vaccine is immunogenic but does not prove that it can prevent the disease (see below).

The true measure for vaccine effectiveness is, however, whether it can prevent the COVID-19 disease or at least protect the vaccinated subject against severe disease. To my knowledge, only one group of scientists, the Oxford group, has included this effectiveness measure in their Phase 1 clinical trial.

The Oxford group's approach may be somewhat risky, as clinical effectiveness measured this way can only be shown if some subjects in both the treatment and the control groups become infected during the trial period. As the number of infected people in some countries is declining, the chance that a test subject may catch the disease may decrease.

There is a risk that only a few individuals in each group will become infected, which would make it difficult to make any meaningful statistical comparison between the groups. To reduce this risk, the Oxford investigators are trying to enroll health care workers, who have a higher risk of becoming infected with COVID-19.

As mentioned, the main purpose of the Phase 1 clinical trial is to demonstrate the safety and tolerance of the vaccine. The participants are therefore observed for any adverse reactions such as local inflammation, irritation, or pain at the site of the injection. A light fever and symptoms of the common cold may also appear. The test subjects in Phase 1 clinical trials are often also observed for changes in their blood chemistry to ensure that the vaccine does not cause any harm to the organs.

Usually, only a limited number of healthy adults are included in a Phase 1 study. Clinical studies done many years back usually only used healthy males as test subjects, but today it is allowable and recommended to also include female test subjects. (The latter must be using an effective contraception in order to participate in the trial.)

Testing Different Doses of the Vaccine

Ideally, a Phase 1 study—or, at the latest, a Phase 2 study—should include vaccination with different doses to see if there is a dose response effect: Does a higher dose result in a better effect?

In Phase 1, where the protection against the COVID-19 disease is not generally measured, a better effect of a higher dose may be a higher level of neutralizing antibodies. In a Phase 2 trial, a better effect may also be measured as a higher level of neutralizing antibodies or a better protection against the COVID-19 disease. The latter would require that several of the participants actually get the disease during the clinical trial. If many test subjects are enrolled, as in the Oxford study (1,112 participants), it may be possible to also test for disease protection in Phase 2.

Testing the Vaccine in Very Young and Older People

Early and late in life, the immune system may behave differently from the way it works in middle-aged adults. It is therefore customary not to include children and very young people in Phase 1 studies. Older people (about 60 years and above) have also been excluded from most Phase 1 trials. This is clearly a limitation for the intended use of any COVID-19 vaccine, as the mortality rate of the COVID-19 infection is at its highest in older age groups.

THE PHASE 2 CLINICAL TRIAL

When the safety of a vaccine candidate has been established in a Phase 1 trial, the sponsor may proceed to the Phase 2 trial. A Phase 2 clinical trial usually includes many more participants than a Phase 1 trial—typically from about 100 to several hundred people.

It is common practice to test the effectiveness of the vaccine in a Phase 2 trial. Ideally, a Phase 2 trial should not only test the vaccine's ability to produce neutralizing antibodies, but also test its ability to protect against the disease. However, of the 16 ongoing trials of COVID-19 vaccine candidates (June 24), only one is testing for disease protection.

As with the Phase 1 study, Phase 2 studies usually only enroll healthy adults as test subjects. However, the age range of the subjects to be enrolled may be broadened. Several of the Phase 2 studies have removed the upper age limit for the enrollment of participants. Whereas most of the Phase 1 studies had an upper age limit for participation at 60 years or less, this upper limit has generally been removed from the Phase 2trials.

PHASE 3 STUDIES

The purpose of a Phase 3 vaccine clinical trial is to assess whether the vaccine is safe in a broad population group. The effectiveness of the vaccine is also assessed. The sponsor generally does not have to show that the vaccine can protect against the disease, although this would be ideal. It's usually enough to show that a vaccine causes the production of neutralizing antibodies in a high percentage of the vaccinated subjects.

However, for COVID-19 vaccine candidates, WHO has recommended that the effectiveness is demonstrated by its ability to reduce the number of those who are infected, severity of the disease, or shedding/transmission of the COVID-19 virus. The vaccine should be effective in at least 50% of the vaccinated subjects.

The safety of the vaccine has been well established before the start of the Phase 3 trial. Participants in younger and older age groups may therefore be included, and the participants do not need to be perfectly healthy. People suffering from chronic diseases, such as diabetes or hypertension, may also be included.

A Phase 3 study usually enrolls several thousand participants and may take years to complete. The Oxford group has applied for the start of a Phase 2/3 study including 10,260 participants (see more details in Chapter 7).

ENHANCED REQUIREMENTS TO MANUFACTURE THE VACCINE

Going from one phase of the clinical trials to the next also means that manufacturing and testing constantly need to be improved.

Requirements to Phase 3 Vaccine Manufacturing

There's generally no significant difference in the requirements regarding the vaccine lots used in Phase 1 and Phase 2 trials. However, the requirements regarding the vaccine material used in Phase 3 trials are much more demanding. For the vaccine material to be used in large-scale Phase 3 studies, regulatory authorities expect the manufacturing processes to be matured, under full control, and validated. The latter means that each process must be demonstrated to work as it is intended to do, and that it works the same way for each new vaccine lot to be manufactured. This may sound like a triviality, but it's often a very complex and resource-demanding task, which may last years. Currently, there is no information regarding whether regulatory authorities would also be willing to cut corners here.

In the previous chapter, we reviewed the many advantages of using an established manufacturing platform. To these advantages, we can add that the use of such well-established platforms would mean that the expensive and time-consuming validation work has already been done.

CUTTING CORNERS IN CLINICAL TRIALS

Regulatory authorities accept that the sponsors and investigators apply for and run more than one clinical trial phase of a COVID-19 vaccine at a time. They are also willing to accelerate the review process for COVID-19 vaccine candidates.

Several sponsors among the 16 front-runners have planned two phases of clinical trials at the same time, for example Phase 1 and Phase 2, or Phase 2 and Phase 3. They have applied for permission to start the next phase before the preceding phase clinical trial has been completed. This may be done if there are sufficient safety data from the preceding trial. This way, any additional risk to the trial participants is minimized. With this approach, the recruitment for the trials, which require many participants (Phase 2 and Phase 3), may be started very early. If needed, for example due to severe adverse events in the preceding trial, the planned subsequent trial may be canceled.

As mentioned above, the requirements to the vaccine lot(s) to be used in Phase 3 studies is much higher than for the lot(s) to be used in Phase 1 or Phase 2 trials. By using a standard manufacturing platform that has already been validated, much time may be saved. Most of the front-running COVID-19 vaccine candidates are based on such standard manufacturing platforms.

AUTHORIZATION TO USE THE VACCINE

The sponsor, usually a pharmaceutical company, applies for permission to market the vaccine when the Phase 3 trials have been successfully completed. Such marketing authorization allows the pharmaceutical company to freely sell the vaccine to all groups for whom the vaccine has been designed.

In an emergency situation such as the current COVID-19 pandemic, it's likely that pharmaceutical companies will not at the beginning apply for full marketing authorization, but rather for restricted authorization. One type of restricted authorization is emergency authorization. This will give the pharmaceutical company the right to sell and distribute the COVID-19 vaccine in an emergency. They may then later apply for full marketing authorization.

KEY TAKEAWAYS

Before a vaccine may be tested in humans for the first time, it usually needs to go through extensive testing in animals.

The animal experiments should show that the vaccine can produce neutralizing antibodies and that it can protect the animals against the infectious disease.

When the vaccine has been shown to be effective in the animal experiments, it must go through a new round of studies to show that it does not harm the animals. These tox studies must usually be completed before the vaccine may be tested in humans. The animal studies usually take up to a couple of years but may be conducted faster.

Regulatory authorities in the US and EU have agreed that animal studies to show that a COVID-19 vaccine candidate is effective are not needed. In addition, they have decided that tox studies may not be needed for all COVID-19 vaccine candidates. If a COVID-19 vaccine is made through the same manufacturing platform as other vaccines, for which the safety has been documented, the tox studies may be skipped. This saves a lot of time.

Testing a new vaccine in humans is done in clinical trials. There are three phases of clinical trials: Phase 1, Phase 2, and Phase 3. Usually, the three phases are done one after the other. To save time, two phases may be initiated at the same time. Several of the COVID-19 vaccine trials are thus Phase 1/2 or Phase 2/3. This also saves a lot of time.

Regulatory authorities, research organizations, and pharmaceutical companies have all shown a willingness to cut corners in the development of COVID-19 vaccines. This means that COVID-19 vaccines may be developed much faster than other vaccines usually are. In the best-case scenario, a COVID-19 vaccine may already become available in the second half of 2020—at least in a limited amount to be used to vaccinate people in high-risk groups (healthcare workers, elderly people, and similar others).

REFERENCES

Bok, K., G. I. Parra, T. Mitra, E. Abente, C. K. Shaver, D. Boon, R. Engle, C. Yu, A. Z. Kapikian, S. V. Sosnovtsev, R. H. Purcell, and K. Y. Green. 2011. "Chimpanzees as an animal model for human norovirus infection and vaccine development." *Proc Natl Acad Sci U S A* 108 (1):325-30.

Cohen, C. 2020. "COVID-19 vaccine protects monkeys from new coronavirus, Chinese biotech reports." Science, Last Modified April 23, accessed June 7. https://www.sciencemag.org/news/2020/04/covid-19-vaccine-protects-monkeys-new-coronavirus-chinese-biotech-reports.

FDA& EMA. 2020. "Summary of FDA & EMA Global Regulators Meeting on Data Requirements Supporting First-in-Human Clinical Trials with SARS-CoV-2 Vaccines." Last Modified March 18, accessed June 7. https://www.fda.gov/news-events/fda-meetings-conferences-and-workshops/summary-fda-ema-global-regulators-meeting-data-requirements-supporting-first-human-clinical-trials.

Lurie, N., M. Saville, R. Hatchett, and J. Halton. 2020. "Developing Covid-19 Vaccines at Pandemic Speed." *N Engl J Med* 382 (21):1969-1973.

Pollard, A. 2020. "A phase 2/3 study to determine the efficacy, safety and immunogenicity of the candidate Coronavirus Disease (COVID-19) vaccine ChAdOx1 nCoV-19." EU Clinical Trial Register, accessed June https://www.clinicaltrialsregister.eu/ctr-search/trial/2020-001228-32/GB.

Revicki, D. A., and L. Frank. 1999. "Pharmacoeconomic evaluation in the real world. Effectiveness versus efficacy studies." *Pharmacoeconomics* 15 (5):423-34.

Rivera-Hernandez T, Carnathan DG, Moyle PM, Toth I, West NP, Young PR, Silvestri G, Walker MJ. . 2014. "The Contribution of Non-human Primate Models to the Development of Human Vaccines." *Discovery Medicin* 18 (101):313-322.

Tacket, SA; Kotloff, KL. 2017. *Initial Clinical Evaluation of New Vaccine Candidate*. Edited by MM Levine, *New Generation Vaccines, 4th. Edition*: CRC Press.

Taylor, NP. 2020. "AstraZeneca's COVID-19 vaccine enters phase 2/3 clinical trial." Fierce Biotech, Last Modified May 22, accessed June 7. https://www.fiercebiotech.com/biotech/astrazeneca-s-covid-19-vaccine-enters-phase-2-3-clinical-trial.

van Doremalen, N; Lambe, T; Spencer, A.; Belij-Rammerstorfer, S. et al. 2020. "ChAdOx1 nCoV-19 vaccination prevents SARS-CoV-2 pneumonia in rhesus macaques." BioRxiv, Last Modified May 13, accessed JUne 7. https://www.biorxiv.org/content/10.1101/2020.05.13.093195v1.

WHO 2020. "WHO Target Product Profiles for COVID-19 Vaccines; Ver. 03." WHO, Last Modified April 29, accessed June 7. https://www.who.int/docs/default-source/blueprint/who-target-product-profiles-for-covid-19-vaccines.pdf?sfvrsn=1d5da7ca_5.

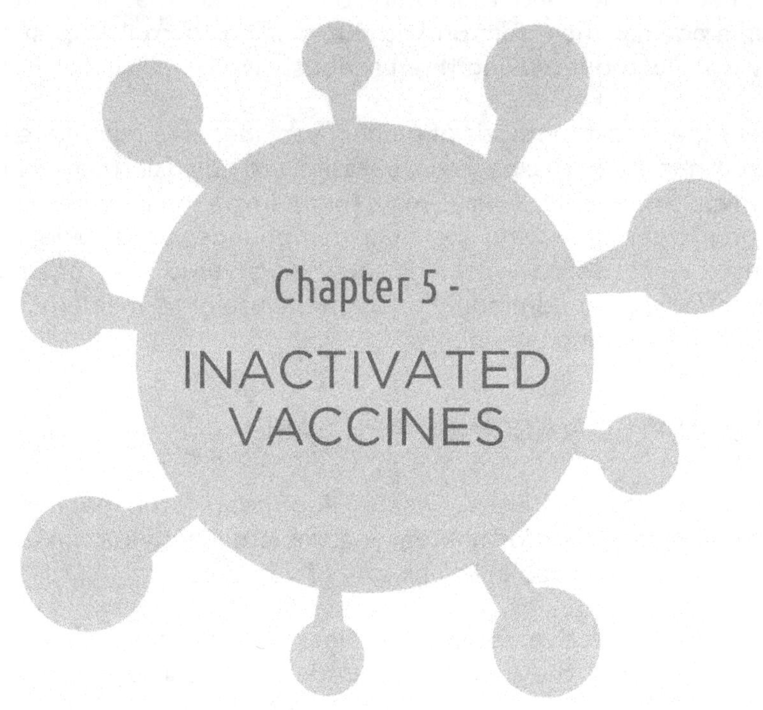
Chapter 5 -
INACTIVATED
VACCINES

When people become infected by a virus, they as a rule become immune to the same virus for a period ranging from some months to many years. The drawback is obviously that they also get sick. A COVID-19 infection may make people seriously ill, and some people may die from the infection.

Because an infection from a live virus can make you seriously ill, we obviously cannot use the live virus in its native form for a vaccination. We need to modify the virus so that it protects people against the infection without making them ill—or, at the very least, without making them seriously ill.

One of the oldest methods of making vaccines is to inactivate the microorganism (virus, bacteria, parasite, etc.) by using physical or chemical treatments. A virus may, for example, be inactivated by heating, treatment with chemical compounds, or radiation. All licensed inactivated vaccines are inactivated by chemical compounds, most commonly through the use of formaldehyde or beta-Propiolactone (see below).

INACTIVATED VACCINES ARE SAFE

Inactivated vaccines are very safe—if, of course, the inactivation is done correctly. Unfortunately, incomplete inactivation of virus vaccines has occurred in the history of vaccines.

Incompletely inactivated virus vaccines have led to outbreaks of the disease that they were intended to protect against. We'll examine one such case below: The Cutter Incident in 1955.

Therefore, inactivation of a virus always needs careful optimization, and the inactivated vaccine needs to be extensively tested. It must be ensured that the inactivation of the virus is complete. This is often done by adding the inactivated virus to various cell types that grow in plastic trays. If there should be any live virus left, the test cells will change form and appear to be sick. In this way, the scientists can find out whether there is any live virus present that could cause the disease. The inactivation is continued until there is no live virus left.

INACTIVATED VACCINES ARE GENERALLY EFFECTIVE

Complete inactivation of the virus is, however, only one side of the coin. The inactivation needs to be complete, but on the other hand, it must also be done in a way that does not damage the parts of the virus that are needed to create an effective immune response. This is most often possible.

As mentioned above, there are several safe and effective inactivated vaccines on the market. As we'll explore below, there is no reason why it should not be possible to develop a safe and effective inactivated vaccine against COVID-19. The development of such vaccines are actually already in good progress.

However, any inactivated vaccine must be evaluated to determine whether the inactivated virus creates an immune response—and also, if possible, whether it offers protection against the disease. This is often done by testing the vaccine in a suitable animal species. A suitable animal species is a species that responds in the same or almost the same way to an infection with the COVID-19 virus as humans (see also Chapter 4). In the late phase of vaccine development in the lab, the efficiency of the vaccines is often tested in rhesus monkeys.

To test whether the vaccine is effective, the animals are first given the vaccine in the same way that a human being would receive it. For example, if a human is going to receive three doses injected into a muscle on days 0, 14, and 28, the tests animals receive the same doses according to the same schedule. The dose may be adjusted for difference in body weight or body surface between the animal test species and humans. A control group is always included so that the scientists can ensure that the protective effect really stems from the vaccine—and not, for example, from the adjuvant.

Thereafter, the animals are infected with the virus. This is called a challenge test. For the COVID-19 virus, this can be done by injecting the COVID-19 virus directly into the monkeys' airways. If the vaccinated animals do not get sick or only get a mild form of the disease, this means that the inactivated vaccine protects the animals against the disease.

THE FIRST SUCCESSFULLY INACTIVATED VACCINE: THE SALK VACCINE

The first successful inactivation of a virus for use as a vaccine was done by the American polio vaccine pioneer Jonas Salk. He used the chemical compound formaldehyde to inactivate the polio virus to be used as a vaccine.

Salk carefully optimized the process so that the polio virus was completely inactivated without harming or destroying the structure of the virus. Inactivation of viruses by use of formaldehyde has since been widely used, and today a number of licensed vaccines inactivated by using formaldehyde are on the market. They include vaccines against poliomyelitis, hepatitis A, and influenza.

Despite Salk's careful work, the use of a formaldehyde-inactivated polio vaccine caused one of the biggest disasters in the history of vaccines.

THE CUTTER INCIDENT

Salk was a scientist working in a lab and could not himself manufacture a sufficient number of polio vaccine doses to vaccinate the many children at risk of getting the polio disease. This task was outsourced to four drug manufacturers, one of which was the Cutter Laboratories. They already had considerable experience in manufacturing other vaccines.

Unfortunately, some of the lots manufactured by the Cutter Laboratories turned out to contain the live polio virus—despite inactivation by formaldehyde. More than 120,000 doses of polio vaccines contained live vaccines. 40,000 children contracted a form of polio that did not result in paralysis. However, 56 children developed paralysis in varying degrees. Five of the vaccinated children died. The vaccine-induced polio outbreak led to an epidemic of polio in which the vaccine-infected children infected others. This second wave of the polio outbreak led to 113 people developing paralysis, and a further five children died.

The Cutter Incident brought the vaccine industry into discredit. It led to a tightening of US regulations for vaccine manufacturing. It also opened the way for litigation against vaccine manufacturers. Probably this and other incidents brought the whole vaccine industry into some disrepute. Even today, many people are skeptical about the safety of vaccines—despite vaccines being some of the safest drugs on the market.

The Cutter Incident illustrates two things of importance for understanding the challenge of bringing a new vaccine such as the COVID-19 vaccine to the market and making it available for the general population.

TAKING A VACCINE FROM THE LAB TO PRODUCTION

First, the vaccine must be safe when manufactured on a lab scale and later when transferred to a proper manufacturing unit capable of making millions of doses. In the race to be the first to bring a COVID-19 vaccine to the market, this fact should never be forgotten. Even though the need for a COVID-19 vaccine is urgent, it is important that the regulations are not relaxed too much. As we'll explore later, it is indeed possible to speed up the development and manufacturing to some extent without sacrificing safety.

Second, the people involved should be aware that transferring a manufacturing process from a lab to a manufacturing unit—or from one manufacturing unit to another—is a difficult matter. Even though a manufacturing process has been carefully described by the scientists who developed the process, some key information may be missing. In addition, the production people (for practical reasons) often have to do things differently from the way the scientists worked.

It is possible to make a decent technical transfer and to test whether all the steps of the processes work as intended, but it requires expertise and takes time. For some of the timelines presented for the COVID-19 vaccine candidates, there seems to be only little time allocated to this task.

SCALING UP THE PROCESS

Closely related to the timelines is the need to scale up the process. Scientists have generally manufactured only a few hundred doses for their initial tests of the vaccines in animals. To make the vaccine available for the first trials in humans, it may be necessary to manufacture several hundred or—for the later phases of clinical trials—several thousands of doses. Compared to manufacturing vaccines for testing in animals, manufacturing vaccines for trials in humans is stringently regulated in most countries. The EU countries have—maybe in contrast to the common perception—the most stringent regulations.

When making an estimate of the time needed to bring a COVID-19 vaccine to the market, all these factors need to be considered, and a proper project plan needs to be developed and followed.

CHEMICAL COMPOUNDS FOR THE INACTIVATION OF VACCINES

During the past years, a number of chemical compounds for the inactivation of vaccines have been developed and tested. However, only two compounds have gained widespread use, namely formaldehyde and beta-Propiolactone.

INACTIVATING VACCINES BY USE OF FORMALDEHYDE

Formaldehyde is often also called formalin. Formaldehyde is the chemical compound itself; it is a gas. Formalin is formaldehyde in water. Formalin contains 37% formaldehyde. Here we'll use the term "formaldehyde."

Formaldehyde Changes the Virus Proteins

Formaldehyde inactivates a vaccine by changing and inactivating the virus proteins. After sufficient long exposure to formaldehyde, the virus loses its ability to infect. However, exposure to formaldehyde may also make the vaccine ineffective by changing or destroying virus proteins that are essential for giving a good immune response in the vaccinated person. As we saw above, the inactivation of a vaccine by formaldehyde therefore needs to be very carefully optimized so that the vaccine is completely inactivated. On the other hand, the inactivation should not be so intensive that the vaccine loses its ability to mount an effective immune response. This is a delicate balance.

Despite a couple of cases many years back, where formaldehyde inactivation went wrong, formaldehyde has successfully been used for the inactivation of a number of vaccines, which are on the market today. The vaccine industry had learned from the past, and today the licensed formaldehyde vaccines are both safe and effective.

INACTIVATING VACCINES BY USE OF BETA-PROPIOLACTONE

A vaccine may also be activated by another chemical compound called beta-Propiolactone. This compound mainly inactivates the vaccine by changing the nucleic acids (the DNA or RNA of the virus). It may also change some of the building blocks (amino acids) of the virus protein, but it rarely leads to the inactivation of the virus proteins or changes them in a way that may lead to an ineffective immune response.

It is simpler and faster to optimize the inactivation of vaccines by using beta-Propiolactone than by using formaldehyde, and inactivation by use of beta-Propiolactone seems to be the preferred method for many new vaccines under development. Once optimized, the inactivation of vaccines also takes only a short time—usually less than 24 hours. Lastly, there is no need to remove any unused beta-Propiolactone, as any beta-Propiolactone left over is rapidly degraded by reaction with water.

The only drawback with beta-Propiolactone is that it is a suspected carcinogenic compound. Hence the handling of beta-Propiolactone necessitates that the technicians and manufacturing operators take appropriate precautions when using beta-Propiolactone. It is important to note that use of beta-Propiolactone to inactivate a vaccine does not expose the people to be vaccinated to any risk of getting cancer. The inactivated vaccine is completely free of beta-Propiolactone.

THE PROS OF INACTIVATED VACCINES

Inactivated vaccines have many advantages. We'll explore the more important ones below.

Inactivated Vaccines Are Very Safe

If inactivated appropriately, inactivated vaccines are among the safest vaccines and most widely applicable of all vaccines.

Inactivated Vaccines Cannot Multiply

Inactivated vaccines contain no live virus and cannot multiply. This means that they can never cause the disease (we're assuming that they have been appropriately inactivated). It also means that they cannot revert to a live virus.

Inactivated Vaccines May Be Given to Pregnant Women

Not all types of vaccines are suitable for the vaccination of pregnant women. However, inactivated vaccines can safely be given to pregnant women. For example, an inactivated flu vaccine may safely be given to a pregnant woman and may offer protection not only to the woman, but also to the baby later on (due to the transfer of antibodies from the mother to the child).

Inactivated Vaccines May Be Given to People With Weakened Immune Systems

Inactivated vaccines may safely be given to people with a weakened or compromised immune response, for example patients suffering from AIDS or cancer.

Testing Inactivated Vaccines Is Less Demanding

Before being released to the public, any vaccine needs to go through a rigorous test program to ensure that it is safe and that it does not contain any unwanted substance such as bacteria, other viruses, DNA from the cells used to grow the virus, etc. An inactivated vaccine does also have to go through most of these tests, but some burdensome tests may not be needed. This may easily save some months when developing the vaccine.

THE CONS OF INACTIVATED VACCINES

In contrast to live viruses and live virus vaccines, inactivated vaccines cannot replicate inside the body. The replication of a virus in the body often gives rise to a strong immune response. Inactivated vaccines may therefore cause a weaker immune response than live attenuated vaccines. Fortunately, there are ways to overcome this potential weakness of inactivated vaccines.

First, we can add a substance to the vaccine—an adjuvant—that enhances the immune response (see also Chapter 4) . One of the most commonly used adjuvants is alum hydroxide. Alum hydroxide is a safe and effective adjuvant that has been used for decades. In recent years, even more effective adjuvants have been developed, and some of these are being used for the development of COVID-19 vaccines, as we will examine in later chapters.

Second, it is possible to enhance the immune response by administering the vaccine more than once. Vaccine scientists obviously always hope and strive to develop a vaccine that needs to be given only once, but sometimes more than one dose needs to be given to get a really effective immune response. The first dose is called the prime dose, whereas the second and any third doses are called booster doses.

When giving more than one dose, the time interval between each dose needs to be carefully optimized. Often, this interval needs to be several months. Of all the ongoing COVID-19 vaccine clinical trials that are using more than one dose, none seems to leave more than four weeks between the first and second dose.

INACTIVATED COVID-19 VACCINES

As we've seen above, one of the simplest ways to develop a new vaccine is to make an inactivated vaccine. Chinese scientists did this a few years back for the development of a vaccine against the EV71 virus that in the Asia-Pacific region causes a polio-like disease. They managed to quickly develop a new vaccine. It is therefore no surprise that four of the COVID-19 vaccine candidates, which are being tested in humans (June 24, 2020), are inactivated vaccines. All of the inactivated COVID-19 vaccines that are currently being tested in humans have been developed and manufactured in China. Below, we'll explore each of these vaccines.

THE SINOVAC COVID-19 INACTIVATED VACCINE: PICOVACC

To develop a COVID-19 vaccine, the Chinese scientists isolated 11 strains of the SARS-CoV-2 virus from patients who had or were having a COVID-19 infection. The patients were from China, Italy, Switzerland, the UK, and Spain. The strains were shown to represent the SARS-CoV-2 virus that circulates and infects people in many different countries.

SELECTION OF THE COVID-19 STRAIN FOR THE VACCINE CANDIDATE

They used one of the strains (CN2) for the COVID-19 vaccine candidate, and the remaining 10 to test the vaccine candidate. They made a viral stock from CN2 and showed that it was pure and stable. Most importantly, they showed that even after 10 generations (replications), only two mutations had occurred. None of these hit the S protein, which is important for mounting neutralizing antibodies.

MANUFACTURING THE COVID-19 VACCINE CANDIDATE

To make large amounts of the COVID-19 virus, they grew the viruses in Vero cells in a standard 50L Cell Factory system (see Chapter 3 for a discussion of the Vero cell line). They inactivated the vaccine by use of beta-Propiolactone and purified it by using three different methods to ensure a pure virus product that meets regulators' requirements. Alum hydroxide was used as adjuvant. From what we have seen above, this is a very traditional approach to the development of an inactivated vaccine.

TESTING THE EFFICACY OF THE PICOVACC VACCINE IN ANIMALS

The COVID-19 vaccine candidate was tested in three animal species: mice, rats, and rhesus monkeys. Mice and rats do not get ill and do not get an illness similar to the disease that humans get. They therefore cannot serve as a model for the human COVID-19 disease. However, vaccination of mice and rats can show whether the vaccine can induce neutralizing antibodies in the COVID-19 S protein, and can give us some useful information about the quality of the antibody response caused by the vaccination.

Testing in Mice and Rats

The mice and rats were injected two times (day 0 and day 7) with four different dose levels (0, 1.5, 3, and 6 micrograms per dose). The 0 micrograms dose obviously served as a control. The vaccination with the COVID-19 vaccine quickly led to a very strong IgG immune response. Already after one week, the mice had on average more than 100 micrograms antibody per milliliter blood. As one microgram is only one millionth of a gram, it may not sound like much, but it is a higher level than what is found in patients successfully recovering from a COVID-19 infection. Although it is well known that one should not conclude too much from the antibody levels achieved in mice and apply them to the levels to be seen in humans, the antibody response observed in the mice indicates that the PiCoVacc COVID-19 vaccine candidate is capable of mounting an antibody response.

Some of the antibodies measured were neutralizing antibodies. These are the types of antibodies that we want because they can prevent the COVID-19 virus from infecting us. The level of neutralizing was only modest after the first week, but rose to 1,500 for the low and medium dose and to 3,000 for the high dose after seven weeks.

The testing of the COVID-19 vaccine in rats produced similar encouraging results. The concentration of neutralizing antibodies reached titers of 2,048 to 4,096 after seven weeks.

Testing in Rhesus Monkeys

Finally, the PiCoVacc inactivated COVID-19 vaccine was tested in rhesus monkeys. Three groups, each with four animals, were used.

One group received saline, and another group received the alum hydroxide adjuvant (the compound used to enhance the immune response, but without the COVID-19 vaccine). These two groups served as controls. The third group received the medium dose (3 micrograms per dose), and the fourth group received the high dose (6 microgram per dose). The animals were vaccinated on days 0, 7, and 7, and thus received the three doses within a short time period.

The day after the third vaccination, the animals were given a large dose of the COVID-19 virus directly into their windpipes. The medium dose seemed to partially protect the animals against getting the COVID-19 disease. The high dose completely protected the animals against the COVID-19 disease. The animals in both vaccinated groups developed neutralizing antibodies. It is, however, unclear whether there was any significant difference between the level reached in the medium- and high-dose group.

Altogether, the PiCoVacc inactivated vaccine seems—based on the animal studies—to be a promising COVID-19 vaccine candidate.

TESTING THE PICOVACC VACCINE IN HUMANS

At the time of writing (June 8), two clinical trials of the Sinovac PiCoVacc vaccine had already been initiated. The inactivated vaccine has been manufactured in Vero cells (Chapter 3). The scientists used alum hydroxide as an adjuvant when they tested the PiCoVacc vaccine candidate in animals. However, the clinical trial protocol does not state that alum hydroxide is being used for the vaccine in the clinical trial.

The First Phase 1/2 Study

The first study plans to recruit 744 participants in the age range of 18 to 59 years in a combined Phase 1/2 study. 144 of the participants will be enrolled in the Phase 1 trial, and 600 in the Phase 2 trial.

Two different vaccination schedules will be tested: an emergency schedule (to be used during the ongoing pandemic) and a routine schedule. All participants will receive two doses. Under the emergency schedule, the test subjects will receive the two doses with a 14-day interval between the doses. In the routine schedule, there will be 28 days between the two doses. Two different doses will be tested.

The participants will be observed for any sign of adverse events such as inflammation or pain at the injection site and for any change in their blood chemistry. The effect of the vaccine will be measured by its ability to generate neutralizing antibodies. The vaccine is considered effective if the level of neutralizing antibodies is equal to or above 8, or if it has increased at least four-fold from the baseline. Whether such a low neutralizing antibodies level (equal to or greater than 8) is really protective remains to be seen. For comparison, the titers in convalescent sera that are used to treat people with the COVID-19 infection is much higher (greater than 160).

No results have been released yet (June 24, 2020). The investigators expect that the last participant will have been vaccinated and tested by August 13, but the monitoring of adverse events continues until December 13, 2020.

The Second Phase 1/2 Study

The second cell line conducted by Sinovac differs from the first clinical trial by including only older adults (age $\geq$ 60 years old). In addition, three different doses instead of two are being tested. The investigators expect that the last participant will have been vaccinated and tested by July 12, but the monitoring continues until July 20, 2021. The clinical trial protocol states that the study will be completed by July 20, 2020, but there is a follow-up visit after 12 months, so it will likely be 2021. No results have been released yet.

THE SINOPHARM COVID-19 INACTIVATED VACCINE

Sinopharm has also initiated two Phase 1/2 clinical trials with two different partners: the Wuhan Institute of Biological Products and the Beijing Institute of Biological Products. The inactivated COVID-19 vaccine has been manufactured in Vero cells (Chapter 3).

THE STUDY DONE WITH THE WUHAN INSTITUTE OF BIOLOGICAL PRODUCTS

The study done in collaboration with the Wuhan Institute of Biological Products will include 1,456 participants split into a large number of groups. The study will include children, younger adults, and older adults. The patients are divided into three age groups: 6–17 years, 18–59 years, and over 60 years. The clinical trial protocol mentions that different doses of the vaccine will be tested, but it does not specify the dose levels to be tested.

The participants will be observed for any adverse events. The investigator will take blood specimens at various time points and examine the specimens for the level of antibodies against the COVID-19 virus. They will also test the T cell response to the vaccine. The vaccine is considered effective if the level of neutralizing antibodies has increased at least four-fold from the baseline.

THE STUDY DONE WITH THE BEIJING INSTITUTE OF BIOLOGICAL PRODUCTS

The design of the study done in collaboration with the Beijing Institute of Biological Products is very similar to the study done with the Wuhan Institute of Biological Products. The major difference is that the former study includes children from three to 17 years old. The investigators will observe the participants and test for vaccine effectiveness in the same way as described for the Wuhan study.

The investigators have not yet reported any results from the two clinical trials in a scientific journal. However, Sinopharm have published several press releases. From these, it appears that the adverse events should be far lower than for other similar products. They do not mention what products they have compared them with. One press release also states that Sinopharm's two manufacturing facilities should be able to deliver 200 million doses of the inactivated vaccine per year.

THE THIRD INACTIVATED VACCINE CANDIDATE FROM CHINA

The WHO "Draft Landscape of COVID-19 Candidate Vaccines" document of June 24 also mentions a third COVID-19 inactivated vaccine from the Institute of Medical Biology, Chinese Academy of Medical Sciences.

The study will enroll 942 participants. They will be divided into eight groups. All groups will receive two doses. Three different dose levels will be tested. Some groups will receive the two doses with two weeks' interval and other groups will receive the doses with four weeks' interval.

The investigators will monitor the participants for any adverse events. They will assess the effectiveness of the vaccine by measuring IgG and neutralizing antibodies to the COVID-19 S protein. They will measure IgM antibodies. In addition, they will measure antibodies to not only the COVID-19 S protein, but also to the N-protein. Last, they will measure T cells response to the COVID-19 virus. This is probably the most comprehensive program for measurement of the immune response to any of the 16 COVID-19 vaccines in clinical trials.

KEY TAKEAWAYS

Inactivated vaccines are very safe. If inactivated correctly, there is no risk at all that the vaccine could cause the disease that it is intended to protect against.

Inactivated vaccines may safely be given to pregnant women and to people with a decreased immune defense, such as those with HIV or cancer.

Inactivated vaccines are usually effective. They rarely mount an immune response that's as effective as a live attenuated vaccine when given as only a single dose without an adjuvant. The immune response generated by an inactivated vaccine can be greatly enhanced by administering more than one dose of the vaccine or by adding an adjuvant to the vaccine.

Inactivated vaccines are easy to develop and manufacture. Several standard platforms for manufacturing exist. Many inactivated vaccines are manufactured in the Vero cell platform (Chapter 3).

Three of the 16 COVID-19 vaccine front-runners, which are in clinical trials, are inactivated vaccines—and all are from China. One of them is being used in two different trials, so there are four trials with inactivated COVID-19 vaccines.

The inactivated vaccines from the two Chinese companies Sinovac and Sinopharm are being tested in Phase 1/2 in a large number of participants. The companies have not yet published any results from the clinical trials in scientific journals. However, Sinopharm have published several press releases. From these, it appears that their inactivated COVID-19 vaccine should be safe and cause few adverse events. They also stated that they should soon be able to manufacture 200 million doses per year.

The vaccine from the Institute of Medical Biology, Chinese Academy of Medical Sciences is in Phase 1 trial

Inactivation of a vaccine is a well-established method to develop a new vaccine. To ensure that it will be effective, more than one dose should be given. It may be an advantage to combine the COVID-19 vaccine with an effective adjuvant. Altogether, it is likely that one or more of the inactivated vaccine candidates may turn out to be safe and effective, and that a substantial number of vaccine doses could be available within a year (mid-2021).

REFERENCES

Barbara Sanders, Martin Koldijk and Hanneke Schuitemaker. 2015. "Inactivated Viral Vaccines." In *Vaccine Analysis: Strategies, Principles, and Control*, edited by B.K. Nunnally et al., 45-80. Heidelberg: Springer-Verlag.

Day, A. 2009. "'An American tragedy'. the Cutter incident and its implications for the Salk polio vaccine in New Zealand 1955-1960." *Health History* 11 (2):42-61.

Delgado, M. F., S. Coviello, A. C. Monsalvo, G. A. Melendi, J. Z. Hernandez, J. P. Batalle, L. Diaz, A. Trento, H. Y. Chang, W. Mitzner, J. Ravetch, J. A. Melero, P. M. Irusta, and F. P. Polack. 2009. "Lack of antibody affinity maturation due to poor Toll-like receptor stimulation leads to enhanced respiratory syncytial virus disease." *Nat Med* 15 (1):34-41.

Delrue, I., D. Verzele, A. Madder, and H. J. Nauwynck. 2012. "Inactivated virus vaccines from chemistry to prophylaxis: merits, risks and challenges." *Expert Rev Vaccines* 11 (6):695-719

Gao, Q., L. Bao, H. Mao, L. Wang, K. Xu, M. Yang, Y. Li, L. Zhu, N. Wang, Z. Lv, H. Gao, X. Ge, B. Kan, Y. Hu, J. Liu, F. Cai, D. Jiang, Y. Yin, C. Qin, J. Li, X. Gong, X. Lou, W. Shi, D. Wu, H. Zhang, L. Zhu, W. Deng, Y. Li, J. Lu, C. Li, X. Wang, W. Yin, Y. Zhang, and C. Qin. 2020. "Rapid development of an inactivated vaccine candidate for SARS-CoV-2." *Science*.

Herrera-Rodriguez, J., A. Signorazzi, M. Holtrop, J. de Vries-Idema, and A. Huckriede. 2019. "Inactivated or damaged? Comparing the effect of inactivation methods on influenza virions to optimize vaccine production." *Vaccine* 37 (12):1630-1637.

Offit, P. A. 2005. "The Cutter incident, 50 years later." *N Engl J Med* 352 (14):1411-2.

Peeples, L. 2020. "News Feature: Avoiding pitfalls in the pursuit of a COVID-19 vaccine." *Proc Natl Acad Sci U S A* 117 (15):8218-8221.

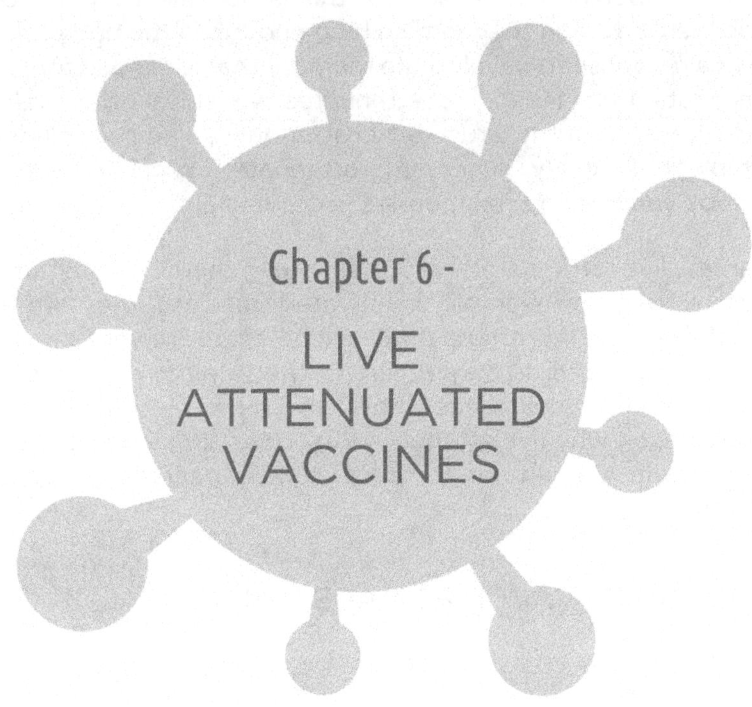

Chapter 6 -
LIVE
ATTENUATED
VACCINES

A live attenuated vaccine is a vaccine that has been made less potent so that it can still infect the host, but without doing as much harm as the wild-type virus. As an example, a live attenuated COVID-19 vaccine would be able to infect human cells and replicate inside those cells, but less effectively than the original wild-type virus.

Live attenuated viruses are known to create a highly effective immune response. The reason for this is because they replicate inside the body, and they remain long enough in the body for the immune response to develop the memory that is needed for long-term protection. Most live attenuated vaccines offer lifelong protection against the virus—often after only a single vaccination. Examples of highly successful attenuated vaccines are the smallpox vaccine and the measles vaccine.

Whereas live attenuated vaccines are generally much more effective than, for example, inactivated vaccines, they are also less safe. For any live attenuated vaccine, there is a very small risk that the vaccine virus may revert to the original wild type and thereby cause severe disease. This is a very rare occurrence, but it's the reason why live attenuated vaccines should not be given to pregnant women or to people with decreased immune function.

ATTENUATED VACCINES MADE BY NATURAL SELECTION

Live attenuated vaccines have contributed significantly to reducing the frequency of or even eradicating serious infectious diseases. As an example, the effective use of the smallpox vaccine has led to the complete eradication of smallpox. Equally, the effective use of the measles vaccine has led to a substantial decrease in the number of measles cases.

Live organisms do mutate, and this also applies to live attenuated vaccines. This means that very rarely, the attenuated virus may revert to a wild-type-like virus that can cause the very disease that the vaccine was intended to protect against. As an example, the oral polio vaccine, which is still in use, may cause paralytic polio disease in about 1 out of 500,000 vaccinated children.

Live attenuated vaccines generally protect the vaccinated individuals against the disease very effectively. In many cases, this protection is lifelong. They are generally considered very safe, but as mentioned, occasionally they may cause the disease that they were meant to protect against.

Why then use live attenuated vaccines instead of inactivated vaccines, or other vaccine types? One reason is because an inactivated vaccine is not always capable of creating an effective immune response in the vaccinated person. As an example, an inactivated measles vaccine used in the past did not prevent the measles disease.

HOW IS A LIVE ATTENUATED VACCINE MADE?

In the past, attenuation of viruses was to a large extent a trial-and-error process. Scientists attempted to grow the virus in organs or cells from other species, and sometimes they were successful. Often, the easily available cells from fertilized hens' eggs (known as chicken embryonic fibroblasts (CEF)) were used. Various groups of scientists were able to grow both measles and vaccines in such cells.

Over time, the viruses became accustomed to growing in these cell types. As part of this process, they lost some of the genes that they formerly used to complete the replication cycle inside human cells or to leave the human cells to infect new cells. In this way, a new strain or subspecies of the virus was created. The modified or attenuated virus is capable of infecting human cells, but cannot replicate itself effectively inside human cells, and generally cannot cause the disease that the original wild-type virus causes.

The major drawback of this approach is that it may take years before scientists succeed in developing an attenuated virus strain that on the one hand replicates well enough to mount an effective immune response and, on the other hand, does not cause the disease. In some cases, it was realized only after the vaccination of humans that a virus had not been sufficiently attenuated.

In the current COVID-19 pandemic, there is unfortunately no time for the natural selection of an attenuated virus strain. Much faster methods for developing a live attenuated vaccine against COVID-19 are needed. Fortunately, such genetic engineering methods exist.

LIVE ATTENUATED VACCINES MADE BY GENETIC ENGINEERING

Methods for the fast development of a live attenuated vaccine have recently been developed. One method, named codon deoptimization, changes the genetic code at several points in the virus genes, whereas another method deletes a single gene or gene region that is needed for the complete virus replication.

At the time of writing (June 11), two COVID-19 vaccine candidates based on codon deoptimization are under development but have not yet entered clinical trials. In addition, a third live attenuated vaccine based on a measles vector is also under development.

A COVID-19 VACCINE MADE BY CODON DEOPTIMIZATION

Below, we are going to look at the codon deoptimization of a COVID-19 vaccine candidate. Before we do that, let's go over some basic genetic-related information again.

GENETIC BACKGROUND

Our genes determine how our body works and how we look. The genes contain the information for making the proteins and molecules that make up our bodies.

The information in our genes is laid down in the genetic code. The code is very simple, consisting of only four letters (these four letters are nucleotides).

In our DNA, the four letters are A, C, G, and T. The genetic code is thus a four-letter code. The information in the genetic code is spelled out in words containing only three letters. There are always only three letters in a genetic code word. Each letter may be A, C, G, or T. Each genetic code word is the code for an amino acid in a protein. Amino acids are the building block of our proteins. Think of a protein as just a long string of amino acids bound together by a special chemical bond called the peptide bond.

Before the information laid down in our DNA code can be used for coding (making) protein, it must be rewritten (transcribed) into another language: the RNA language. The RNA language also consists of four letters, but one letter is different: A, C, G, and U. As we can see, the T has been replaced by a U. As it is the RNA in the form of messenger RNA (mRNA) that directly codes for the proteins that our cells make, the genetic code is shown as an RNA code—even though our genes are made of DNA. The process of rewriting the RNA code to a protein code is called translation. To sum up, the genetic information in DNA is transcribed to the RNA code, which is then translated into a protein code.

It can be calculated that the genetic code contains 64 code words. Each of the three letters in an RNA code word may thus be either A, C, G, or U (remember, it is an RNA code). This gives us 4 x 4 x 4 = 64 different words. A code word may, for example, be AAA, CCC, GGG, or UUU, but mixtures of the letters are equally possible. Examples of code words are GAG, GGC, AAC, ACG, and CAU.

The genetic code is universal. This means that all live organisms use the same code, but in some organisms, the genetic information is stored in DNA genes, whereas in others it is stored in RNA genes. In many viruses, including the COVID-19 virus, the genes are made of RNA. Other RNA viruses are polio, hepatitis C, and measles. Viruses may also store their genetic information in DNA. Examples of DNA viruses are Hepatitis B, human papillomavirus (that may cause cervix cancer), and common-cold adenoviruses.

The genetic code contains 64 code words, whereas our proteins consist of only 20 different words or amino acids. This means that there could be more than one code word for each amino acid. In fact, this is the case. Four of the code words in the genetic code have special functions, such as starting (one code word) or ending (three code words) the translation from the RNA language into the protein language. This leaves 60 code words for only 20 amino acids. This means that it is often possible to exchange one letter for another—for example, an A for a G—without necessarily changing the protein. This fact is the key to understanding how "code deoptimization" may be used to create viruses that look identical to the original (wild-type) virus but that do not replicate nearly as well in human cells as the original virus. We'll explore this below.

CODON DEOPTIMIZED LIVE ATTENUATED VACCINES

When a virus like the COVID-19 virus replicates, sometimes changes in the code occur. We call these changes mutations. A mutation can be a change of just one letter of the code to another, for example from C to U. This does not need to change the amino acid in the virus protein. As an example, the four RNA code words GCU, GCC, GCA, and GCG are all codes for the same amino acid alanine. As we can see, it doesn't matter what the last letter is. The code message remains the same.

THE GENES IN RNA VIRUSES MUTATE QUITE OFTEN

The genes in RNA viruses mutate quite often, as they are missing the proofreading function that is found in DNA replication. Many mutations are so simple that they consist of exchanging just one of the four letters for another letter. As we have seen, there are often several code words for the same amino acid of the protein, so a mutation does not necessarily lead to a protein or virus that is different from the existing one. Such mutations are called silent mutations.

In situations where more than one genetic code word can code for the same amino acid, one would expect that each of the possible code words occur with the same probability. One would also expect that pairs of different codes would occur equally often. However, this is not the case.

THE CODE HAS BEEN OPTIMIZED TO PRODUCE THE STRONGEST VIRUS

In recent years, scientists have discovered that some genetic code words—coding for a particular amino acid—occur more frequently than they should (if all code words had the same chance of coding for a particular amino acid). This "abnormality" is even more pronounced for a pair of code words.

The reason for this is not fully known. However, scientists speculate that the code in the course of evolution has been optimized to ensure that the existing viruses are those that can best replicate themselves.

They therefore studied what happens if they change the code so that it still codes for the same proteins and hence still produces the same virus, in this case the COVID-19 virus. This has not yet been studied in any detail for the COVID-19 virus, but it has been done for a number of other similar viruses.

DEOPTIMIZATION OF THE CODE LEADS TO AN ATTENUATED VIRUS

When the code is changed, the virus may still be able to infect and replicate in human cells. However, when the code has been deoptimized in this way, the new virus may not be able to replicate as effectively as the original virus. But to the immune system, the two viruses look identical. The antibody response generated after vaccination with the modified virus will protect equally well against the original wild-type virus.

It is therefore possible in a lab to create a new virus type, which will produce the same immune response as the original virus, but which will be highly attenuated and incapable of causing disease—or only capable of causing a much milder disease than the original virus. This genetic engineering, which is called codon deoptimization, makes possible the rapid development of a live attenuated virus.

At the time of writing (June 24), no live attenuated vaccine is being tested in humans. There are three COVID-19 vaccine candidates in "preclinical evaluation." Preclinical evaluation is a broad concept. It means that some testing of the vaccine candidate has begun, but it doesn't tell us anything about how far the scientists have come. Preclinical evaluation ranges from very early lab experiments in "test tubes" to elaborate studies in monkeys.

Three COVID-19 live attenuated vaccine candidates are in preclinical evaluation. Two of those are based on the codon deoptimization approach that we reviewed above. Below, we'll look more at one of the COVID-19 vaccine candidates, which is based on this type of genetic engineering.

THE CODAGENIX COVID-19 VACCINE

Codagenix is a US company that has worked with codon deoptimization for several years. The company has six human vaccines in its pipeline. One of these, a universal flu vaccine CodaVax-H1N1, has been tested in a clinical trial. The company has not presented the results of the trial yet. Prior to the clinical trial, Codagenix had shown that its flu vaccine candidate provided protection against influenza in mice and ferrets.

The flu vaccine CodaVax-H1N1 went into clinical trial as early as February 2017, and the clinical trial was completed in September 2018. The trial was designed to assess the safety and effectiveness of the vaccine. To assess whether the flu vaccine candidate was effective, the investigators measured antibodies in blood specimens from the vaccinated subjects. To my knowledge, the results of the clinical trial have not been reported yet. This means that we do not know whether the Codagenix vaccine candidate is safe and effective in humans.

Codagenix is now applying the same platform as it used for its flu vaccine candidate to develop a COVID-19 vaccine candidate. It is a whole live attenuated vaccine and targets not only the COVID-19 spike protein, but also a number of other proteins in the capsule and envelope. This time, Codagenix is collaborating with the Serum Institute of India—the world's largest vaccine manufacturer. The Codagenix COVID-19 vaccine candidate is, as mentioned, in preclinical trial. We therefore don't yet know whether this approach to developing a live attenuated vaccine will work.

KEY TAKEAWAYS

Live attenuated vaccines have been shown to be highly effective. A live attenuated vaccine is probably the most effective vaccine type known. A single dose often gives lifelong protection against the disease. They are also generally very safe. However, in very rare cases, they may cause the disease that they were meant to protect against.

The live attenuated vaccines on the market today have all been developed by natural selection, through which they have been grown in a cell line other than their natural host. The development of a live attenuated vaccine by natural selection may, however, take many years.

In the current COVID-19 pandemic, there is no time for the development of COVID-19 live attenuated vaccines by natural selection. Instead, scientists must rely on genetic engineering.

One such approach is codon deoptimization. Through this method, the genetic code is changed without changing the virus proteins. Therefore, to the immune system, a vaccine made by codon deoptimization looks exactly like the original wild-type virus. However, it replicates less effectively and is generally very safe. No live attenuated vaccine based on codon deoptimization—or other similar genetic engineering techniques—has made it to the market yet, but the approach looks promising.

REFERENCES

Codagenix. 2020. "Our technology." Codageneix Inc., accessed June 30. https://codagenix.com/technology/platform-overview/.

Groenke, N., J. Trimpert, S. Merz, A. M. Conradie, E. Wyler, H. Zhang, O. G. Hazapis, S. Rausch, M. Landthaler, N. Osterrieder, and D. Kunec. 2020. "Mechanism of Virus Attenuation by Codon Pair Deoptimization." *Cell Rep* 31 (4):107586.

Konopka-Anstadt, J. L., R. Campagnoli, A. Vincent, J. Shaw, L. Wei, N. T. Wynn, S. E. Smithee, E. Bujaki, M. Te Yeh, M. Laassri, T. Zagorodnyaya, A. J. Weiner, K. Chumakov, R. Andino, A. Macadam, O. Kew, and C. C. Burns. 2020. "Development of a new oral poliovirus vaccine for the eradication end game using codon deoptimization." *NPJ Vaccines* 5:26.

Lauring, A. S., J. O. Jones, and R. Andino. 2010. "Rationalizing the development of live attenuated virus vaccines." *Nat Biotechnol* 28 (6):573-9.

Meng, J., S. Lee, A. L. Hotard, and M. L. Moore. 2014. "Refining the balance of attenuation and immunogenicity of respiratory syncytial virus by targeted codon deoptimization of virulence genes." *mBio* 5 (5):e01704-14.

Mueller, S., C. B. Stauft, R. Kalkeri, F. Koidei, A. Kushnir, S. Tasker, and J. R. Coleman. 2020. "A codon-pair deoptimized live-attenuated vaccine against respiratory syncytial virus is immunogenic and efficacious in non-human primates." *Vaccine* 38 (14):2943-2948.

Stauft, C. B., C. Yang, J. R. Coleman, D. Boltz, C. Chin, A. Kushnir, and S. Mueller. 2019. "Live-attenuated H1N1 influenza vaccine candidate displays potent efficacy in mice and ferrets." *PLoS One* 14 (10):e0223784.

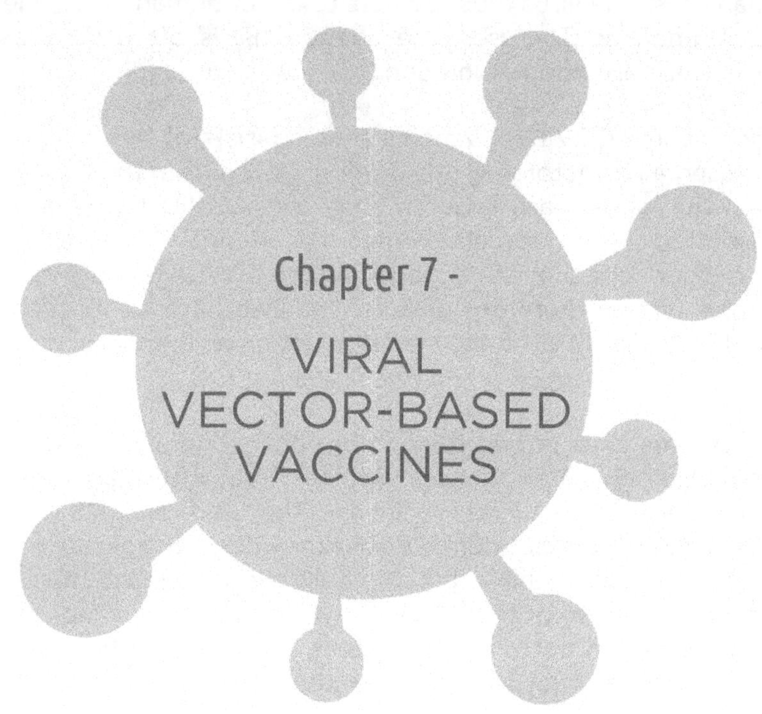

Chapter 7 -
VIRAL
VECTOR-BASED
VACCINES

The title of this chapter may sound a little complicated because it uses scientific jargon. However, here the word "vector" has nothing to do with mathematics or physics. The term is used in biology and genetics to refer to a mechanism to transfer genes from one cell into another.

Here we'll define a vector as a virus (different from the COVID-19 virus) that is used to transport one or more COVID-19 genes into human cells. The virus must be able to infect human cells. One of the common cold viruses, the adenovirus, is often used as a vector. It is very good at infecting us.

A viral vector COVID-19 vaccine thus consists of two parts: the virus used as a vector and one or more genes from the COVID-19 virus. The virus part ensures that the COVID-19 genes are transported into our cells. When the COVID-19 genes have entered our cells, they start producing the COVID-19 proteins. Our immune system therefore believes that we have been infected with the COVID-19 virus and starts mounting an immune response against it.

Viral vectors exist in two forms: non-replicating and replicating. Non-replicating viral vector vaccines are often also called replication-deficient viral vaccines. The non-replicating viral vectors can only infect our cells, but they cannot replicate inside the cells. When they have infected our cells, they make their own proteins and those of the COVID-19 virus. In contrast, replicating viral vectors can both infect our cells and replicate themselves. Non-replicating viral vectors are thus similar to inactivated vaccines, whereas replicating viral vector vaccines are more like live attenuated vaccines.

Below, we'll explore non-replicating viral vector vaccines. Currently (July 2) there are no replicating viral vector vaccines in clinical trials, but 17 such vaccines are under development. However, for the sake of brevity, we won't review those vaccine candidates here.

NON-REPLICATING VIRAL VECTOR VACCINES

Non-replicating viral vector vaccines can easily infect cells, but they cannot replicate themselves inside the cells, and they cannot cause disease. A person vaccinated with an adenovirus vector COVID-19 vaccine neither catches the common cold as a result of the vaccination—even though the adenovirus was used as a vector—nor contracts the COVID-19 disease. Non-replicating viral vector vaccines are therefore very safe, similar to inactivated vaccines.

Non-replicating viral vector vaccines do have a few drawbacks. To mount a strong immune response, the dose usually has to be high compared to the dose needed for a replicating viral vector vaccine. In addition, a prime dose and one or two booster doses may be required to create a strong and long-lasting immune response. A way to further boost the immune response is to use one viral vector for the prime dose and another for the booster dose(s). This approach has been successfully used to make a vaccine against Ebola.

VIRAL VECTOR VACCINES ARE MADE BY GENETIC ENGINEERING

Non-replicating viral vector vaccines are made by genetic engineering. Genetic engineering just means that the scientists take out one or more genes and replace them with the genes that they want to get into the human cells. They may take out the virus genes that are needed for the virus to replicate inside human cells. This way, they get a non-replicating viral vector. Alternatively, they may modify some of the virus genes so that the virus' ability to replicate is reduced. They then get a replicating viral vector.

A popular virus for making non-replicating viral vector vaccines is the common cold virus adenovirus 5, often abbreviated as Ad5. The adenovirus has the same form of genetic material as we have, namely a double-stranded DNA (just much smaller). The adenovirus can be made into a non-replicating vector by removing its E1 genes (see details below).

TYPES OF ADENOVIRUS VIRAL VECTORS

There exist many different adenoviruses that infect us and give us the common cold. Many of us have been infected with adenovirus type 5 (Ad5). As a result, many of us have antibodies against the Ad5 virus. In America, about 40%–50% of humans have neutralizing antibodies against Ad5; in China, it is about 75%; and in other Asian countries and in Africa, it is even higher.

When a person has neutralizing antibodies against adenovirus 5, there is a risk that a vaccine based on this vector may not work well. Binding of the neutralizing antibody to the adenovirus-based vaccine may prevent the vaccine from infecting our cells and hence from generating an effective immune response. Although this may not happen the first time a person is vaccinated, it may happen if a second dose is needed.

Other adenoviruses, for example adenovirus 26 (Ad26), only rarely infect us and may be more suitable as a viral vector, because only a few of us have antibodies against Ad26. For this reason, some scientists prefer to develop vaccines based on Ad26. It is also possible to use an adenovirus from one of our closely related species: apes, such as the chimpanzee.

ADENOVIRUS 5 VIRAL VECTORS

Adenovirus 5 has been used extensively as a viral vector in making viral vector vaccine candidates for more than 30 years. Despite the potential disadvantage of using Ad5, discussed above, it remains the most popular viral vector platform for the development of vaccines, including vaccines against the COVID-19 virus. The COVID-19 vaccine candidate from the Chinese company CanSino Biologics, which has advanced to a Phase 2 clinical trial, is thus based on the Ad5 viral vector. Other COVID-19 vaccine candidates in the preclinical phase are also based on the Ad5 viral vector.

ADENOVIRUS 26 VIRAL VECTORS

To avoid the potential pitfalls of using the Ad5 viral vector, some scientists as mentioned prefer to work with other adenoviruses—for example, Ad26. While some of us may have caught the common cold or an eye infection caused by adenovirus 26 in the past, far fewer of us have antibodies against Ad26 than against Ad5. A reduced immune response is therefore less likely for an Ad26 vector vaccine than for an Ad5 vector vaccine.

CHIMPANZEE VIRAL VECTORS

The adenoviruses that we have reviewed above are often called human adenoviruses. This means that they can infect humans, which also means that there exists a group of adenoviruses called non-human adenoviruses. Some of these may infect our close relatives, such as chimpanzees, orangutans, and gorillas.

Scientists working at the University of Oxford's Jenner Institute are using a chimpanzee adenovirus vector to develop vaccines against COVID-19 and other viruses. The Oxford group has developed a chimpanzee viral vector named ChAdOx1, which they are using for the development of a COVID-19 vaccine.

Outside Africa, only a few people (0%–4%) have antibodies against chimpanzee adenoviruses, whereas up to 30% in certain areas of Africa may have such antibodies. Therefore, by using this chimpanzee viral vector, the risk of getting a less effective immune response is low (outside Africa). We'll explore the ChAdOx1 vaccine candidate later in this chapter.

MAKING A NON-REPLICATING VIRAL VACCINE

Scientists make an adenovirus incapable of replicating by cutting out the E1 genes of its DNA. Without the E1 genes, the adenovirus cannot replicate itself. Often, the scientists also cut out another gene (or gene region): the E3 gene. This is mainly done to create more space to insert other genes, such as some COVID-19 genes, but also to avoid the E3 genes modifying the immune response in an unfavorable way.

After the unwanted adenovirus genes have been cut out, the desired genes—for example, the genes expressing the COVID-19 spike proteins—are inserted into the adenovirus DNA. They are inserted in the form of a "cassette." The cassette contains genes other than the COVID-19 genes that ensure that the production of the proteins coded for by the inserted COVID-19 genes becomes very effective.

As a result of the genetic engineering, the adenovirus vector can now infect human cells (as it could before) and start making its own proteins *and* the foreign proteins (here the COVID-19 spike proteins).

However, the adenovirus vector cannot complete its life cycle inside the human cells. Hence, no new adenovirus vectors can leave the infected cell, and the infection cannot spread from cell to cell. As a result, a non-replicating virus vector can at most infect the same number of cells as the number of virus vectors in a dose. As an example, if one dose contains 10 billion virus vectors, only up to 10 billion human cells may be infected. This may limit the strength of the immune response.

PRODUCER CELL LINES

Before we can use a non-replicating viral vector as a vaccine, we must be able to grow it—make more copies of it—so that we can make large amounts of the vaccine. The next question is: How can a non-replicating vaccine grow? The answer is that it can in fact grow, but only in certain cell types that have themselves been genetically engineered. Such cell types are called producer cells; they supply the factors that the non-replicating viral vector vaccine needs. (We reviewed the commonly used producer cells lines, the HEK293 cell line and the PER.C6 cell line, in Chapter 3.)

COVID-19 VIRAL VECTOR VACCINE CANDIDATES

There are many different viral vector COVID-19 vaccine candidates under development; as of June 9, there were 34 such candidates. Of the non-replicating vaccine candidates, four were already in clinical trials as of June 30. One—the CanSino Biologics (China) vaccine—is in Phase 2, and the other—from the University of Oxford's Jenner Institute (the UK)—is in Phase 2/3. Just as I was completing the editing of this book, the Russian Gamaleya Research Institute announced that they had initiated clinical trials with two adenoviral COVID-19 vaccines. One is based on the Ad5 virus and the other on the Ad26 virus.

As these four vaccine candidates are among the front-runners in the COVID-19 race, we are going to discuss them in some detail below.

ADENOVIRUS VECTOR VACCINES

As mentioned above, the adenovirus vector platform has been in use for more than 30 years and is seen as being a most promising technology. Vaccines based on this platform have not been approved for general use and hence have not made it to commercial large-scale manufacturing.

The Chinese company CanSino Biologics has, however, developed an Ad5-based vaccine against Ebola. The vaccine candidate was tested in Phase 2 studies. Based on these studies, the Chinese authorities approved it for emergency use against Ebola in China without undergoing a Phase 3 trial. The reason given was that the Ebola epidemic at that time had died out, so it would not have been possible to demonstrate that the vaccine could protect against Ebola in a Phase 3 trial. CanSino Biologics has stated that they can manufacture 70 million doses of an Ad5 viral vector vaccine.

A Phase 3 trial of another Ebola vaccine (Ad26.ZeBov/MVA-BN-Filo), partly based on the Ad26 platform, has been completed. The company developing this vaccine, Janssen Pharmaceutical Companies (part of Johnson & Johnson), has filed for licensure of the vaccine. The prime dose contained the Ad26 vaccine, whereas the booster doses contained the MVA-BN-Filo vaccine, developed by Bavarian Nordic. If it is approved, it should be noted that this is not a "pure" adenovirus vaccine in the sense that the booster dose was made by a different technology. This means that there still wouldn't be any approved (licensed) vaccine on the market based solely on the adenovirus vector technology. This is not meant to cast a shadow over adenovirus viral vector vaccine candidates; it's simply a reminder that despite the current enthusiasm for adenovirus-based vaccines, they have yet to prove their value.

THE CANSINO BIOLOGICS VACCINE CANDIDATE

One of the lead candidates in the COVID-19 vaccine race is the CanSino Biologics Ad5-based vaccine. Although it has already completed Phase 1, the results have not yet been published (June 12). However, as all studies of new vaccines have to be announced in a clinical trial database, we do have some knowledge about both the completed Phase 1 trial and the yet-to-begin Phase 2 trial. The information about the Phase 1 and Phase 2 trials has been published in the Chinese Clinical Trial Register.

THE PHASE 1 AD5 COVID-19 VACCINE TRIAL

In the Phase 1 trial, the test subjects had to be between 18 and 60 years old. The Phase 1 trial was an open trial (see Chapter 4). The trial did not include any control subjects. The trial included 36 people in each group (low, middle, and high dose). The purpose of the Phase 1 trial was to test three different doses of the COVID-19 adenovirus vector vaccine, and to see whether the test subjects got any adverse effects. The three doses tested were 50 billion viruses, 100 billion viruses, and—according to the published information—100 billion viruses. As we can see, the same amount is stated for both the middle dose and high dose, which means that the 100-billion-virus figure for the high dose is probably a typo.

For the sake of clarity, here one billion is to be understood as an American billion: 1,000,000,000. (In Europe, one billion is 1,000,000,000,000.)

During the trial, the test subjects were observed for adverse effects. At different time points, blood specimens were drawn to test for antibodies against the COVID-19 spike proteins (S proteins). The formation of antibodies against the S protein is the desired effect of a COVID-19 vaccine, as antibodies against the S protein may protect the vaccinated person from getting the COVID-19 infection (see also Chapter 3).

The Chinese scientists measured IgG antibodies and neutralizing antibodies against the S protein. As mentioned, we do not yet have access to these data yet, but apparently the outcome of the

Phase 1 trial must have been satisfactory, as the Chinese investigators decided to move on with a Phase 2 trial.

THE PHASE 2 AD5 COVID-19 VACCINE TRIAL

In the Phase 2 trial, no upper age limit has been set. 500 test subjects will be enrolled, and the trial will include a control ("placebo") group. The control group does not receive the vaccine but an injection with a similar-looking fluid. The trial will be blinded so that no one knows whether a subject gets the vaccine or the control injection before the study has been completed. Of the 500 test subjects, 250 will get the middle dose, 125 will get the low dose, and 125 will get a control (placebo) dose.

As in the Phase 1 trial, the scientists will look for any sign of adverse effects and measure IgG antibodies and neutralizing antibodies against the COVID-19 S protein. They will also, as in the Phase 1 trial, test for the formation of neutralizing antibodies against adenovirus 5.

Apparently, the trial has not started recruiting test subjects yet (June 12). The trial itself lasts six months, and thereafter statistics and reporting will have to be done, so it is unlikely that we will know the results before the end of 2020.

THE CHIMPANZEE VACCINE

A group of scientists at the University of Oxford have since 2012 worked with a chimpanzee adenovirus viral vector, which today is named ChAdOx1, and have made several vaccine candidates based on this vector. Most importantly, they have tested a vaccine against another coronavirus, MERS, in both rhesus monkeys and humans.

In the trial with rhesus monkeys, they found that a single dose of the ChAdOx1-based vaccine produced a strong immune response against MERS, and that the vaccine protected the rhesus monkeys against injury of the airways and prevented severe infection of the lungs (pneumonia).

In the trial of the MERS vaccine in humans, the scientists tested three different doses: five billion, 25 billion, and 50 billion viral particles per dose. They found that all three dose levels were safe. The test subjects experienced only minor adverse effects such as short-lived fever. All dose levels produced an immune response in most of the participants. In the group receiving the high dose, all nine participants had IgG antibodies 28 and 56 days after the vaccine. In the subjects who showed up for a follow-up visit one year after the vaccination, five out of six still had IgG antibodies against the MERS vaccine.

Only one of the five participants receiving the low dose developed neutralizing antibodies. None of the eight participants receiving the middle dose produced neutralizing antibodies. In the high-dose group, four of the nine participants made neutralizing antibodies. All participants in all three dose groups mounted a T-cell immune response against MERS. The titer of the neutralizing antibodies was low and did not exceed 16. The titer of neutralizing antibodies needed to protect against MERS or COVID-19 is not yet known. However, for the use of convalescence serum to treat severely ill patients with the COVID-19 disease, the FDA recommends that the titer should be 160, or at least 80. So, a titer equal to or less than 16 appears to be low.

The positive results of the ChAdOx1-based MERS vaccine tests in rhesus monkeys and humans make the ChAdOx1 COVID-19 vaccine candidate an interesting candidate—even though only four of nine participants given the high dose developed low levels of neutralizing antibodies. In the section below, we'll take a closer look at the ChAdOx1-based COVID-19 vaccine candidate.

THE CHADOX1 COVID-19 VACCINE CANDIDATE

Using a similar approach to the one used for the development of the ChAdOx1-based MERS vaccine candidate, the scientists at Oxford in collaboration with other researchers have developed a COVID-19 vaccine candidate.

The vaccine has been tested in a mouse model for the COVID-19 disease and, more importantly, in rhesus monkeys. The results were, in a preliminary form, just published when I drafted this chapter in mid-May. I do not expect the final paper to deviate from the draft version with regard to the results of the study. Here, we'll only look at the results from the vaccination of the rhesus monkeys.

Six monkeys were vaccinated with 25 billion ChAdOx1 COVID-19 virus particles. This is half of the dose being used for the trial of the ChAdOx1-based vaccine candidate that is currently being tested in humans (see below). They only got a single dose. All six animals developed IgG antibodies and neutralizing antibodies against COVID-19. Three monkeys served as the control group and were vaccinated with another ChAdOx1-based vaccine.

To test whether the vaccination actually protected the animals against a COVID-19 infection, the animals were exposed to COVID-19 viruses. The viruses were administered in the windpipe (trachea), nose, eye, and mouth. The animals vaccinated with the ChAdOx1 COVID-19 vaccine candidate did better and recovered faster than the animals in the control group, but they did get infected. However, most importantly, none of the animals in the group vaccinated with the COVID-19 vaccine candidate showed any sign of severe lung infection (pneumonia)—the dreaded complication of the COVID-19 infection in humans.

THE FIRST CHADOX1 COVID-19 VACCINE CLINICAL TRIAL

The ChAdOx1 COVID-19 vaccine candidate is being tested in humans. The scientists at Oxford have named the vaccine candidate ChAdOx1 nCoV-19.

THE OXFORD GROUP STRIVES TO PROVE THAT THE VACCINE PROTECTS AGAINST THE COVID-19 DISEASE

The design of this trial may be risky compared to the other trials of currently ongoing (June 24) COVID-19 vaccine candidates, as the investigators will test the vaccine's ability to protect against the COVID-19 disease. This means that some of the test subjects need to catch a COVID-19 infection "in real life" to see whether the vaccine is effective. The other trials measure the effectiveness of the vaccine candidate by measuring antibodies in blood specimens from the vaccinated subjects. There is therefore no need for the subjects to become infected with the COVID-19 virus.

Containment Measures Reduce the Number of Infected People

Due to the measures taken to prevent the spread of COVID-19 in the UK, where the Oxford trial is taking place, the number of people infected per day is constantly decreasing. The number of new cases in the UK was 6,111 as of May 6; 2,711 as of May 18; and 1,266 as of June 12. There are about 66 million people in the UK. Using the latest number of deaths per day available, we can calculate that about two out of 100,000 (1,266/66,000,000) will get the COVID-19 infection each day.

Altogether, 1,112 people will be enrolled according to the latest trial protocol update. The participants will be divided into four groups. Most of the participants will get only one dose of the vaccine, whereas one group will get a prime dose and a booster dose. It has not been published how many subjects will be in each group. If we assume that about 60% of the trial participants will get the ChAdOx1 COVID-19 vaccine and use the round number 1,100 for enrollment, 660 will be given the COVID-19 vaccine—and 440 will get the control vaccine.

Will There Be Enough Infected People to Show That the Vaccine Protects Against the Disease?

The trial runs for six months with an option for the test subjects to visit again after one year. This means that each subject will be monitored for at least six months (roughly 200 days). Each day, each subject will have a two in 100,000 chance of becoming infected with COVID-19 (see above). During the trial period, the total risk of being infected will be 200 times: 2/100,000 or 0.004. This means that about three out of 660 trial participants in the vaccine group might become infected in the six-month trial period.

In a similar way, we can calculate that about two people of the 440 participants in the control groups would be infected. I do not have access to the statistical calculations behind the design of the trial, so the above example is only an attempt to provide a simplified estimate. It is, however, clear that due to the steadily declining number of COVID-19 infections per day in the UK, only a few people in each group would become infected during the six-month trial period. This might make it difficult to see whether the COVID-19 vaccine candidate protects against the disease. When the trial was designed back in April, many more people were becoming infected per day, and it would likely have been possible to see whether the vaccine protects against the COVID-19 disease. Possibly to compensate for the decreasing number of infected people per day, the Oxford investigators plan to enroll participants with a higher risk of getting infected—for example, healthcare workers. The investigators are also monitoring the development of antibodies against the COVID-19 S protein and the development of a T-cell response. This will make it possible to evaluate whether the vaccine is immunogenic even if there won't be sufficient data to show that it protects against the COVID-19 disease.

The Oxford group has teamed up with the big pharma company AstraZeneca to be able to scale up the manufacturing of their vaccine candidate. AstraZeneca aims to have 30 million vaccines ready in September 2020. Given that the results of the Phase 1/2 trial might not be available at that time, it is difficult to see how an approved (licensed) vaccine could be available at that early stage. It is, however, possible that the UK health authorities might permit the emergency use of the COVID-19 vaccine without having data from a Phase 3 trial.

THE PHASE 2/3 CHADOX1 COVID-19 VACCINE TRIAL

In the Phase 2/3 trial, the Oxford investigators plan to enroll 10,260 subjects, of whom 60 will be below 18 years old, 10,000 will be between 18 and 59 years old, and 200 will be more than 60 years old. The investigators will, as in the Phase 1/2 trial, evaluate whether the vaccine protects against the disease. They will also measure IgG, neutralizing antibodies, and T-cell response against the COVID-19 S protein.

THE J&J ADENOVIRUS 26 VECTOR VACCINE

Currently (June 12), no adenovirus 26 vaccine candidate is being tested in humans. However, Janssen Pharmaceutical Companies has previously developed an Ebola vaccine candidate based on an adenovirus 26 viral platform—to be used together with the MVA-BN-Filo as a booster (see earlier in this chapter).

Although this adenovirus-26-based vaccine candidate has not yet entered clinical trials, it's worth mentioning because it is based on an existing platform capable of making millions of doses. The platform consists of Janssen Pharmaceutical Companies' AdVac® and PER.C® technologies. The AdVac® technology is used to make an adenovirus-based COVID-19 vaccine candidate. The PERC.6 cell line is used to manufacture the COVID-19 vaccine candidate.

Janssen Pharmaceutical Companies is owned by Johnson & Johnson, which has entered into a partnership with the Biomedical Advanced Research and Development Authority (BARDA). BARDA and Johnson & Johnson have together committed more than one billion USD of investment to co-fund vaccine research, development, and clinical testing. Such a massive commitment to an established vaccine platform would increase the chance of developing a vaccine.

J&J stated that they expect to start clinical trials no later than September 2020, and they expect that the first batches authorized for emergency use might be available in early 2021. Their ambition is to be able to supply one billion doses worldwide for emergency use. No timeline for the availability of this number of doses has been given.

THE GAMALEYA RESEARCH INSTITUTE AD5 AND AD26 VACCINES

Just as I finished editing this book (June 24, 2020), two other non-replicating adenoviral COVID-19 vaccines entered clinical trials. The vaccines have been developed by the Gamaleya Research Institute in Moscow, Russia.

At the time of writing, only sparse information about the vaccines was available. However, from the clinical trial protocol, it appears that investigators will test two different non-replicating adenoviral vaccines. One is based on the Ad26 virus and the other on the Ad5 virus. Both types contain the gene for the COVID-19 S protein.

Two groups of participants will receive only one dose of either the Ad26-based or the Ad5-based vaccine. The third group will receive two doses of the vaccines. The first will be the Ad26-based vaccine and the second will be the Ad5-based vaccine.

The investigators will monitor the participants for any adverse effects. They will also measure IgG and neutralizing antibodies against the COVID-19 S protein as well as T cells against the S protein.

The trial will include 38 people. According to the protocol, it began on June 17, 2020, and will end on August 15, 2020.

KEY TAKEAWAYS

Above, we have seen that there are several promising adenovirus-based vaccine candidates in development.

CanSino Biologics has completed a Phase 1 trial with their adenovirus-5-based COVID-19 vaccine candidate and has started a Phase 2 trial with the vaccine candidate. They have stated that they can manufacture 70 million doses. No time period for this was given, but it is presumably meant to be per year. While this would be impressive, there would still be a long way to go to make enough doses for true mass vaccination.

The scientists at the Jenner Institute have started Phase 1/2 and Phase 2/3 trials with their ChAdOx1-based COVID-19 vaccine candidate. They expect to have results from the first group(s) of participants as early as June 2020. The Oxford group has teamed up with AstraZeneca to increase their manufacturing capacity. AstraZeneca have stated that they will make 30 million doses available by September 2020. Given that the results of the Phase 1/2 trial might not be available by that time, it is difficult to see how an approved (licensed) vaccine could be available at that early date. Possibly, AstraZeneca may succeed in obtaining emergency-use authorization in the UK.

Just as I finished editing the book, AstraZeneca announced that they had agreed with the EU to deliver up to 400 million doses of this vaccine to EU countries.

The Gamaleya Research Institute entered clinical trial with their Ad5 and Ad 26 COVID-19 vaccines. Besides testing the two vaccines individually, there are testing them in a two-dose scheduled with the Ad26 vaccine as prime vaccination and the Ad5 vaccine as booster vaccination. This approach may enhance the immune response.

The J&J Ad26 COVID-19 vaccine candidate has not entered clinical trials yet. However, J&J has shown that they can manufacture a large number of doses based on their technology.

Altogether, it is likely that one or more non-replicating viral vector COVID-19 vaccines will be available in 2020—at least for emergency use.

REFERENCES

AstraZeneca. 2020. "AstraZeneca and Oxford University announce landmark agreement for COVID-19 vaccine." Last Modified April 30, 2020, accessed May 20. https://www.astrazeneca.com/media-centre/press-releases/2020/astrazeneca-and-oxford-university-announce-landmark-agreement-for-covid-19-vaccine.html.

Enjuanes L, Zuñiga S, Castaño-Rodriguez C, et al. 2016. "Molecular Basis of Coronavirus Virulence and Vaccine Development." *Advances in Virus Research* 96.

Folegatti, P. M., M. Bittaye, A. Flaxman, F. R. Lopez, D. Bellamy, A. Kupke, C. Mair, R. Makinson, J. Sheridan, C. Rohde, S. Halwe, Y. Jeong, Y. S. Park, J. O. Kim, M. Song, A. Boyd, N. Tran, D. Silman, I. Poulton, M. Datoo, J. Marshal, Y. Themistocleous, A. Lawrie, R. Roberts, E. Berrie, S. Becker, T. Lambe, A. Hill, K. Ewer, and S. Gilbert. 2020. "Safety and immunogenicity of a candidate Middle East respiratory syndrome coronavirus viral-vectored vaccine: a dose-escalation, open-label, non-randomised, uncontrolled, phase 1 trial." *Lancet Infect Dis*.

Guo, J., M. Mondal, and D. Zhou. 2018. "Development of novel vaccine vectors: Chimpanzee adenoviral vectors." *Hum Vaccin Immunother* 14 (7):1679-1685..

Hodges, B. L., H. K. Evans, R. S. Everett, E. Y. Ding, D. Serra, and A. Amalfitano. 2001. "Adenovirus vectors with the 100K gene deleted and their potential for multiple gene therapy applications." *J Virol* 75 (13):5913-20.

Humphreys, I. R., and S. Sebastian. 2018. "Novel viral vectors in infectious diseases." *Immunology* 153 (1):1-9.

Johnson & Johnson. 2020. "Johnson & Johnson Announces a Lead Vaccine Candidate for COVID-19; Landmark New Partnership with U.S. Department of Health & Human Services; and Commitment to Supply One Billion Vaccines Worldwide for Emergency Pandemic Use."

Korber B, Fischer WM, Gnanakaran S, Yoon H, Theiler J, Abfalterer W, Foley B1, Giorgi EE, Bhattacharya T, Parker MD3, Partridge DG, Evans CM, Freeman TM, de Silva TI, LaBranche CC, and Montefiori DC. 2020. "Spike mutation pipeline reveals the emergence of a more transmissible form of SARS-CoV-2." Last Modified May 5, 2020, accessed May 23. https://www.biorxiv.org/content/10.1101/2020.04.29.069054v2.full.pdf.

Lowe, Dereak. 2020. "In the Pipeline. A close look at the frontrunning coronavirus vaccines as of May1." Last Modified May 15, 2020, accessed May 18. https://blogs.sciencemag.org/pipeline/archives/2020/04/23/a-close-look-at-the-frontrunning-coronavirus-vaccines-as-of-april-23.

Marley, S. 2020. "AstraZeneca Aims for 30 Million U.K. Vaccine Doses by September." Bloomberg, Last Modified May 17, 2020, accessed May 20.

https://www.bloomberg.com/news/articles/2020-05-17/astrazeneca-aims-for-30-million-u-k-vaccine-doses-by-september.

TrialSiteNews. 2020. "CanSino Biologics' Ad5-nCoV the First COVID-19 Vaccine to Phase II Clinical Trials." Last Modified Apr 19, 2020, accessed May 20. https://www.trialsitenews.com/cansino-biologics-ad5-ncov-the-first-covid-19-vaccine-to-phase-ii-clinical-trials/.

University of Oxford. 2020. "A Study of a Candidate COVID-19 Vaccine (COV001)." Last Modified May 19, 2020. https://clinicaltrials.gov/ct2/show/NCT04324606?term=vaccine&cond=covid-19&draw=2.

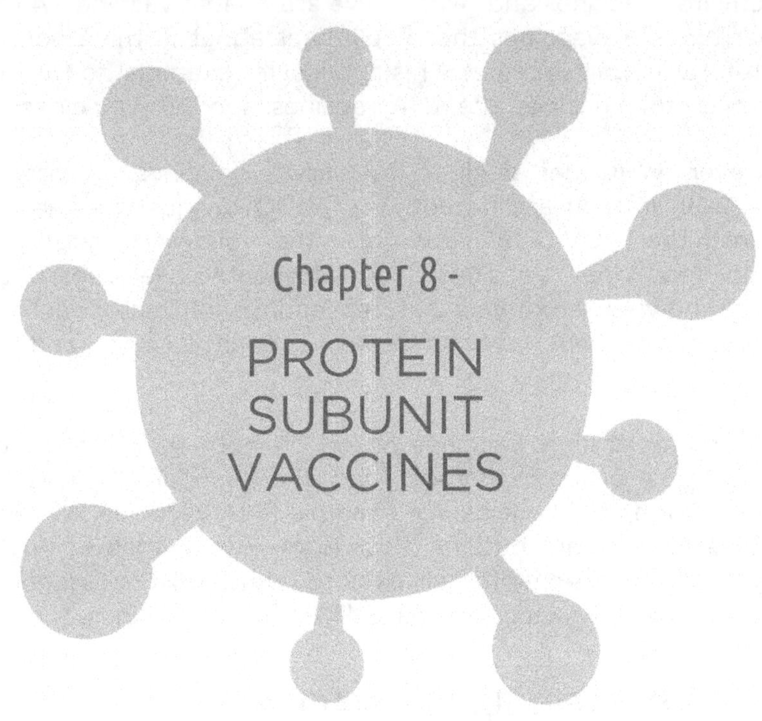
Chapter 8 -
PROTEIN
SUBUNIT
VACCINES

A subunit vaccine may be defined as a vaccine that targets only a part of the virus instead of the whole virus. We may define a virus subunit vaccine as a vaccine that includes only parts of the virus instead of the entire virus.

You could therefore say that all vaccines that are not directed against the whole virus are subunit vaccines. The only types of vaccines that would then not be subunit vaccines would be whole inactivated vaccines and (whole) live attenuated vaccines. All the other types of vaccines that you'll hear about in this book are therefore subunit vaccines. This applies, for example, to the viral vector-based vaccines, the RNA vaccines, and DNA vaccines.

However, WHO has decided to classify vaccines against the COVID-19 virus in a different way. WHO divides the vaccines against the COVID-19 virus into the following categories: inactivated virus vaccines, live attenuated vaccines, non-replicating viral vector vaccines, replicating viral vector vaccines, RNA vaccines, DNA vaccines, protein subunit vaccines, and VLP vaccines.

WHO thus classifies vaccines based on both their target (the whole virus or part thereof) and the technology used for manufacturing the vaccine, for example RNA vaccines. This may not seem logical, but in this book, we'll follow WHO's classification. This chapter will explore two of WHO's categories: protein subunit vaccines and virus-like particle vaccines.

MAKING PROTEIN SUBUNIT VACCINES

The term "protein subunit vaccine" clearly indicates that these vaccines consist of one or more proteins. Proteins to be used as vaccines may be made by different methods.

Most often, they are made using recombinant technology, which we'll learn more about below. Essentially, one or more genes from the COVID-19 virus are inserted into another organism such as the bacterium *E. coli*, the baculovirus, or another organism that then produces the COVID-19 protein(s). A protein that is made by inserting foreign genes into an organism is called a recombinant protein. This term simply indicates that the genes have been combined in a new way.

The important difference between protein subunit vaccines and, for example, viral vector vaccines is that for the former, the production of the COVID-19 proteins takes place outside the human body. The protein is harvested from the cell culture and used as a vaccine. Only the protein itself is injected.

Instead of using live cell cultures to make the proteins, they may also be made directly by chemical synthesis in a machine that connects the amino acids to produce the right protein. However, this technology is unsuitable for making proteins consisting of many amino acids and is rarely used for making vaccines.

Protein subunit vaccines are very popular. When I finished editing this chapter (June 24), three protein subunit vaccines were being tested in humans, and about 50 other protein subunit vaccines were being developed. This figure does not include the virus-like particle vaccines (see below).

COVID-19 VIRUS PROTEIN SUBUNIT VACCINES

An advantage of COVID-19 subunit vaccines is that they can target a very specific part of the COVID-19 virus. Most COVID-19 protein subunit vaccines target the spike protein (S protein). As mentioned earlier (Chapter 1), the S protein has a pivotal role in the binding of COVID-19 viruses to human cells and in infecting the human cells. One part of the large S protein binds to the ACE2 receptor on the human cells. This is the first step in infecting our cells. A vaccine that targets the S protein or a part thereof, for example the ACE2 Receptor-Binding Domain, can prevent an infection from the COVID-19 virus.

VACCINES AGAINST SUBUNITS OF THE S PROTEIN

It's possible to make subunit vaccines that only target part of the S protein. The S protein can be divided into two subunits: S1 and S2. The S1 subunit is responsible for binding to the ACE2 receptor on the human cells, whereas S2 is responsible for the fusion of the COVID-19 virus membrane and the human cell membrane. It is possible to make a COVID-19 vaccine that targets only the S1 subunit of the S protein. It's also possible to make a vaccine that targets an even smaller part of the S protein, namely the receptor-binding domain (RBD)—the part of the S protein that binds to the ACE2 receptor.

VIRUS-LIKE PARTICLE COVID-19 VACCINES

At the other end of the spectrum, it is also possible to make a subunit vaccine that consists of the whole "shell" of the COVID-19 virus. These types of vaccines are called virus-like particles (VLP). VLPs are similar to whole inactivated virus vaccines in the sense that they present the whole surface of the virus to the immune system. However, they do not contain the COVID-19 virus RNA, so they cannot multiply or replicate inside the human cells. They are one of the safest types of vaccines because they do not contain the genetic information: the RNA. They therefore cannot cause the disease that they are designed to protect against. When I edited this chapter (June 24), there was no virus-like particle COVID-19 vaccine in clinical trial, but several such vaccines were under development.

CHEMICAL SYNTHESIS OF THE VACCINE PROTEIN

The simplest method to make a protein subunit vaccine would be, at least theoretically, to directly make the target protein—for example, the S protein—by chemical synthesis in a machine. This is an automated process, and it doesn't require the use of any live cells or components from animals. It uses the 20 amino acids (in a modified form) that are found in proteins in live organisms and assembles them according to the instruction it has: the sequence of the different amino acids. Using the instruction and the modified amino acids, it synthesizes the requested protein. A protein subunit vaccine made by chemical synthesis is a very safe vaccine.

However, the S protein is a long protein that contains more than 1,200 amino acids. This makes it impossible with today's technology to produce the whole COVID-19 virus S protein by chemical synthesis. The upper limit for such chemical synthesis is generally considered to be less than 100 amino acids, although a few peptides longer than this have been successfully synthesized. It may, however, be possible to synthesize smaller parts of the S protein, such as the Receptor-Binding Domain.

There was no chemically synthesized protein subunit in any clinical trial when I edited this chapter (June 24). However, there seems to be a few such COVID-19 vaccine candidates under development among the more than 125 known candidates, which are not yet in clinical development.

RECOMBINANT SYNTHESIS OF THE VACCINE PROTEIN

Another method to make a subunit vaccine would be to synthesize a part of the virus's protein by using recombinant technology. A recombinant protein might sound very complicated, but its process is actually quite simple. Essentially, the scientists insert the genes coding for the wanted protein(s) into the DNA or the RNA of another organism: the host organism. When the host organism multiplies, it produces not only its own proteins, but also the COVID-19 virus proteins, for which the genes have been inserted into the host organism's DNA or RNA.

Many common biological drugs—for example, human insulin for the treatment of diabetes—are manufactured by using recombinant technology. Monoclonal antibodies used for the treatment of immunological diseases—such as multiple sclerosis and cancer—are also made by recombinant technology.

Recombinant proteins may be produced in many different organisms. The bacterium *E. coli* was very popular in the early days of recombinant technology, but today other host organisms are becoming more popular. Human insulins from Novo Nordisk are often made with yeast cells (*Saccharomyces cerevisiae*). There seems to be no COVID-19 vaccine candidate in development that's made in *E. coli* or a yeast cell. In the vaccine industry, manufacturing protein subunit vaccines and virus-like particles in baculovirus and insect cells is becoming increasing popular.

MANUFACTURING VACCINES IN INSECT CELLS

With this technology, the gene of interest—for example, the gene coding for the COVID-19 S protein—is inserted into a virus, the baculovirus, that infects insect cells. Inside the insect cells, the baculovirus produces its own proteins and the COVID-19 S protein. When the manufacturing of the spike protein has been completed, the S protein can be harvested from the insect cells and used as a vaccine.

THE BACULOVIRUS INSECT CELL MANUFACTURING PLATFORM

You may not have heard about the baculovirus before. However, many years back, it was used as a biological pesticide—for example, in private gardens. The baculovirus is a relatively large DNA virus that only infects insect cells. A given baculovirus does not infect all types of insects but only one or a few species. This makes it possible to use the baculovirus specifically for preventing insect diseases that cause damage to, for example, cabbage. However, our interest here is not in pesticides for cabbage, but in the use of the baculovirus for making protein subunit vaccines.

The baculovirus usually infects the insect in its worm stage. One type of baculovirus infects the fall armyworm (*Spodoptera frugiperda*). For more than 30 years, scientists have used cells from the armyworm to make proteins. They grow the baculoviruses in a culture of the insect cells, from which they can harvest the protein that they are interested in. Several cell lines have been established from the fall armyworm. One of them, the Sf9 cell line, is popular for making recombinant proteins.

This platform for manufacturing proteins, including virus subunit vaccines, is called the insect cell baculovirus expression system in the field of science. Here, we'll call it the baculovirus platform.

Today the baculovirus platform is as equally well established as a manufacturing platform for vaccines as some of the other platforms that we've learned about in this book: the Vero cell and the PER.C6 cell line. The first human vaccine to be manufactured and licensed on this platform was a vaccine against human papillomavirus (HPV)—a virus that may cause cervical cancer. This vaccine was licensed in 2007 in the EU and in 2009 in the US under the name Cervarix®.

The baculovirus platform is a versatile platform that may be used to manufacture proteins and subunit vaccines, including virus-like particles. The baculovirus contains about 155 genes, of which about 50 are not needed for its ability to replicate inside insect cells. This means that a large number of foreign genes may be inserted into a baculovirus.

THE NOVAVAX NANOPARTICLE VACCINE NVX-COV2373

Novavax have been making recombinant proteins for several years. They use Sf9 cells and the baculovirus to produce vaccine candidates. They have developed a technology that they can use to make recombinant nanoparticles. Novavax have two vaccine candidates in Phase 3 clinical trials and are also developing a COVID-19 protein subunit vaccine: the Novavax Nanoparticle Vaccine NVX-CoV2373. This vaccine candidate is currently being tested in humans in a Phase 1/2 clinical trial.

The Novavax COVID-19 vaccine has been manufactured in the baculovirus platform by inserting the COVID-19 virus genes for the S protein into the baculovirus DNA. To get the baculovirus to manufacture the whole S protein, the genes for the whole S protein were inserted. The recombinant protein is therefore named a full-length S protein.

You may recall that the COVID-19 virus is an RNA virus. You may therefore wonder how S proteins can be made by a DNA virus such as the baculovirus. This is simply done by transcribing the COVID-19 virus RNA genes to a DNA code and then inserting the DNA genes into the baculovirus. This way, the baculoviruses will produce the COVID-19 virus S proteins in the insect cells that they infect.

TESTING THE NOVAVAX NVX-COV2373 VACCINE IN BABOONS

Novavax have tested some of their earlier vaccine candidates and the COVID-19 vaccine candidate in baboons. They have summarized their findings in the PowerPoint presentation: "NVX-CoV2373 vaccine for COVID-19" (May 13, 2020). They found that the antibody response in baboons for their Ebola vaccine candidate predicted the response in humans.

The protein subunit vaccine CoV2373 binds strongly to the human ACE2 receptor. It is therefore expected that the NVX-CoV2373 vaccine will produce antibodies that prevent the COVID-19 virus from binding to the ACE2 receptor and hence from infecting human cells.

In baboons, vaccination with the NVX-CoV2373 vaccine in combination with the Matrix-M adjuvant resulted in the production of high levels of neutralizing antibodies. The best response was seen after two doses of the high-concentration vaccine (25 micrograms). As Novavax have previously shown that the level of neutralizing antibodies found in baboons can predict the antibody response in humans, there is hope that the NVX-CoV2373 vaccine will be effective in humans.

THE NOVAVAX CLINICAL TRIALS

Novavax have already begun clinical trials with their COVID-19 subunit vaccine candidate. The title of their clinical trial application is "Evaluation of the Safety and Immunogenicity of a SARS-CoV-2 rS (COVID-19) Nanoparticle Vaccine With / Without Matrix-M Adjuvant."

The title tells us that the purpose of the study is to evaluate whether the vaccine candidate is safe and effective in the sense that it can mount an immune response in the vaccinated person. It also informs us that they're going to use a nanoparticle to get the S protein into the cells. Lastly, it tells us that they're going to use an adjuvant called Matrix-M. The latter is quite interesting because the Matrix-M adjuvant is a new adjuvant developed by

Novavax. Novavax state that the Matrix-M adjuvant promotes a strong immune response, and that it stimulates the production of both T1 and T2 cells, as well as all classes of antibodies.

Novavax plans to enroll 130 participants in an age group of 18 to 59 years old. The participants are divided into five groups:

- One group will be a controlled group (placebo), in which the participants are only given a saline injection. All participants will receive two injections with a three-week interval in between.

- The second group will receive 25 micrograms of the subunit vaccine without the adjuvant.

- The third and fourth groups will receive either five micrograms or 25 micrograms of the subunit vaccine with or without the Matrix-M adjuvant.

- The fifth group is quite interesting. The participants will receive 25 micrograms of the subunit vaccine with or without the Matrix-M adjuvant as a prime dose. However, the "booster dose" will only be saline as a placebo. This group has obviously been included to see whether a booster dose is needed at all.

The participants will as usual be observed for adverse events such as local inflammation and pain or fever. According to the protocol, the scientists will measure the IgG antibody level in blood specimens to see whether the vaccine is effective. Apparently, they do not plan to measure neutralizing antibodies. The study was scheduled to start on May 25 and is planned to run until December 31, 2020, when the last participant has been evaluated. However, Novavax expect to be able to present the first results from the trial in July 2020. They have stated that they will apply for emergency-use authorization and that production could be scaled up to 100 million doses by the end of 2020.

Novavax have also planned a Phase 2 clinical trial. It has not been registered in the clinical trial databases yet, but it has been briefly described in the PowerPoint presentation: "NVX-CoV2373 vaccine for COVID-19." It will basically follow the same protocol as used for the Phase 1 clinical trial described above, but will enroll 2,200 participants, of whom 1,000 will be older adults.

THE CLOVER BIOPHARMACEUTICALS COVID-19 VACCINE

Clover Biopharmaceuticals is a Chinese company. Their COVID-19 vaccine is a protein subunit vaccine consisting of a trimer of the COVID-19 S protein. "Trimer" is just a name for a protein consisting of three identical protein units. The trimer consists of three S protein units. The COVID-19 S protein exists as a trimer on the surface of the virus, so a protein subunit vaccine consisting of a trimer of the S protein mimics the natural S protein.

The title of the clinical trial is: "A Phase 1, Randomized, Double-blind, Placebo-controlled, First-in-human Study to Evaluate the Safety and Immunogenicity of SCB 2019, a Recombinant SARS-CoV-2 Trimeric S Protein Subunit Vaccine for COVID-19 in Healthy Volunteers."

The title tells us that the COVID-19 vaccine is made by recombinant technology but does not specify how the subunit vaccine was made. The company's homepage does not give us more information. However, it tells us that they have made no changes to the S protein, so it is exactly the same as the S protein on the surface of the COVID-19 virus. They also inform us that they will be able to manufacture up to 100 million doses per year.

The trial is conducted in collaboration with GSK and Dynavax. The study will enroll 150 participants that will be divided into 15 groups.

The investigators will study two different dose levels: three micrograms and 30 micrograms. They will test the subunit vaccine with and without two different adjuvants. The first adjuvant is the ASO3 developed by GSK. This has been used in several other vaccines made by GSK.

The second adjuvant is actually a mixture of two different adjuvants: the CpG 1018 adjuvant and aluminum hydroxide. The

CpG 1018 adjuvant has been developed by Dynavax. It stimulates the native immune system. The combination of the CpG 1018 adjuvant and the aluminum hydroxide should produce a strong immune stimulation.

The investigators will monitor the participants for any adverse effects. They will also measure IgG and neutralizing antibodies.

THE ANHUI ZHIFEI LONGCOM BIOPHARMACEUTICAL COVID-19 VACCINE

Anhui Zhifei Longcom Biopharmaceutical is a Chinese company that has developed several vaccine candidates. Their COVID-19 subunit vaccine was approved for entering clinical trials by the Chinese authorities just the day before I finished editing this book (June 24, 2020).

Only sparse data about the vaccine was available. From the WHO draft landscape of COVID-19 vaccines as of June 24, 2020, it appears that it is a recombinant vaccine consisting of a dimer of the COVID-19 S protein's receptor-binding domain. This means that it targets a small part of the S protein—but exactly the part that the COVID-19 S protein uses to enter our cells. The clinical trial protocol had not been published when I finished editing the book (June 24, 2020).

KEY TAKEAWAYS

Protein subunit vaccines consist of one or more proteins. Most COVID-19 protein subunit vaccines target the COVID-19 spike protein. There are more than 50 COVID-19 protein subunit vaccines in development, in which the virus-like particle vaccine candidates are included.

Protein subunit vaccines may be made by using chemical synthesis or recombinant technology. The COVID-19 S protein is a large protein containing more than 1,200 amino acids. Due to its size, the S protein cannot be chemically synthesized. Therefore, all COVID-19 protein subunit vaccine candidates in development are made by recombinant technology.

The baculovirus platform is a popular and well-established platform for making protein subunit vaccines. Novavax have used the baculovirus platform to manufacture their COVID-19 vaccine candidate: the NVX-CoV2373 Vaccine. The vaccine is administered together with the Matrix-M adjuvant. The vaccine has been shown to produce a strong neutralizing antibody response in baboons.

This vaccine is being tested in a Phase 1 trial enrolling 130 participants. A Phase 2 trial—enrolling 2,200 participants, including 100 older adults—has been planned. Novavax have stated that they expect to be able to manufacture 100 million doses this year.

Just when I finished editing the book, two other protein subunit vaccines entered clinical trials.

One was developed by the Chinese company Clover Biopharmaceuticals. It is a trimer of the COVID-19 S protein. The S protein on the surface of the COVID-19 virus is present in the form of a trimer, S protein vaccination with this subunit vaccine should mimic the natural infection.

The other protein subunit vaccine was from the Chinese company Anhui Zhifei Longcom Biopharmaceutical It targets a narrow part of the S protein, namely the Receptor Binding Domain.

All three protein subunit vaccines have been developed by experienced vaccine developers. Protein subunit vaccines are generally very safe and often provide a reasonably strong immune response, so there is hope that one or more of these candidates will be successful.

REFERENCES

Abdulrahman, W., L. Radu, F. Garzoni, O. Kolesnikova, K. Gupta, J. Osz-Papai, I. Berger, and A. Poterszman. 2015. "The production of multiprotein complexes in insect cells using the baculovirus expression system." *Methods Mol Biol* 1261:91-114. doi: 10.1007/978-1-4939-2230-7_5.

Corradin, G., A. V. Kajava, and A. Verdini. 2010. "Long synthetic peptides for the production of vaccines and drugs: a technological platform coming of age." *Sci Transl Med* 2 (50):50rv3.

Demotz, S., C. Moulon, M. A. Roggero, N. Fasel, and S. Masina. 2001. "Native-like, long synthetic peptides as components of sub-unit vaccines: practical and theoretical considerations for their use in humans." *Mol Immunol* 38 (6):415-22.

Gleen, G. 2020. "NVX-CoV2373 Vaccine for COVID-19." Last Modified May 13, accessed May 23. https://novavax.com/download/files/2020-05-13WVCWebinarCOVID19v3.pdf.

Mena, Ja, Kamen AA. 2011. "Insect Cell Technology Is a Versatile and Robust Vaccine Manufacturing Platform." *Expert Reviews of Vaccines* 10 (1):1063-1081.

Novavax. 2020. "Evaluation of the Safety and Immunogenicity of a SARS-CoV-2 rS (COVID-19) Nanoparticle Vaccine With/Without Matrix-M Adjuvant." Last Modified May 15, accessed May 23. https://clinicaltrials.gov/ct2/show/NCT04368988?term=vaccine&recrs=a&cond=covid-19&draw=2&rank=10.

O'Shaughnessy, L., and S. Doyle. 2011. "Purification of proteins from baculovirus-infected insect cells." *Methods Mol Biol* 681:295-309.

Strobl, F., S. M. Ghorbanpour, D. Palmberger, and G. Striedner. 2020. "Evaluation of screening platforms for virus-like particle production with the baculovirus expression vector system in insect cells." *Sci Rep* 10 (1):1065. doi: 10.1038/s41598-020-57761-w.

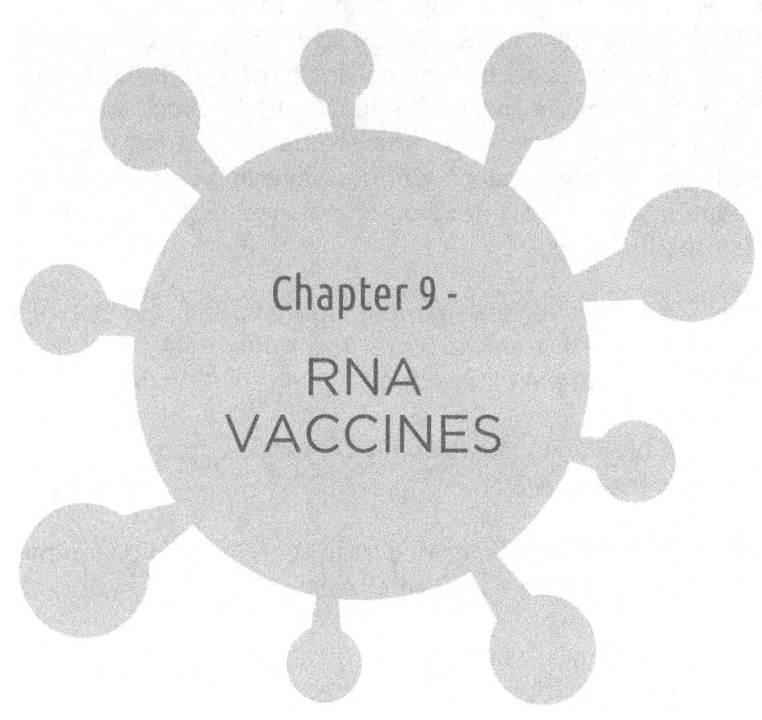
Chapter 9 -
RNA
VACCINES

Vaccines based on RNA is a relatively new invention, and no vaccine RNA vaccine has up to now been licensed for commercial use. Compared to traditional vaccines, such as inactivated and attenuated vaccines, the manufacturing of RNA vaccines is simple. The RNA itself may be produced in large amounts without the need for any host cells. It is much cheaper to manufacture RNA vaccines than more traditional vaccines.

There is therefore great hope that RNA vaccines against the COVID-19 virus will be successful, so that it will be possible to make millions or even billions of doses of a COVID-19 vaccine within a short time frame. Of the 16 COVID-19 vaccine candidates in clinical trials as of June 24, four are based on RNA technology. In addition, at the time of writing, several other RNA vaccine candidates were being developed but had not yet entered the human-testing phase.

Below, we'll first briefly review some basic genetic-related information. We'll then explore the four RNA vaccine lead candidates that are in clinical trials:

- The LNP-encapsulated mRNA vaccine from Moderna/NIAID

- The four mRNA vaccines from BioNTech / Fosun Pharma / Pfizer (called 3 LNP-mRNA)

- The LNP-nCoVsaRNA mRNA candidate from Imperial College London

- The CureVac mRNA vaccine

The vaccine names may sound complicated, but the technology behind the names is in principle quite simple. LNP stands for lipid nanoparticles—a technology or method used to get the messenger RNA into human cells. All four companies use this technology to get the mRNA into the cells.

GENETIC BACKGROUND

In our cells, the genetic information is stored in DNA. When our cells want to make a protein, they first have to transcribe the information coded in the DNA into another genetic code: the RNA code. Before the protein synthesis can start, the information stored in the DNA will thus have to be transcribed to RNA.

RNA is a nucleic acid like DNA. Each DNA code word contains three letters. Any letter can be A, C, G, or T. Each RNA code word contains the same three letters as the DNA—namely A, C, and G—but in RNA, the fourth letter in the DNA code word is replaced by a U. However, the information in the two languages of RNA and DNA is identical. This means that when you know the DNA code, you also know the RNA code—and the other way around.

DNA is a double strand (a double helix). When the DNA code is transcribed to the RNA code, the DNA double strand opens up, and the RNA code is made as a copy of the DNA code. The only difference is that the letter T in the DNA is replaced with the letter U in the RNA. Even though the genetic information is stored in the DNA, the genetic code is usually presented as an RNA code. As an example, the code that codes for the first amino acid in a protein is written as the RNA codeword AUG—not as ATG as it would be in the DNA code.

There are several forms of RNA in our cells, but only one carries the genetic code. This type of RNA is called the messenger RNA (mRNA). It tells the cell's protein synthesis machinery how to assemble the amino acids so that the right protein is made. The idea behind mRNA vaccines is that a piece of mRNA injected directly into our cells will trick the cells into making the protein that mRNA codes for.

Two other types of RNA are involved in protein synthesis in our cells. One is ribosomal RNA (rRNA), on which the protein synthesis takes place. The other is the transfer RNA molecules that bring the amino acid building blocks to the rRNA. However, we won't delve into rRNA or tRNA in this book.

THE COVID-19 VIRUS MAKES MRNA IN OUR CELLS

In contrast to our cells, the coronavirus does not contain any DNA at all. It contains a special form of RNA. When a coronavirus enters a human cell, it starts replicating itself by making more copies of its RNA. Then the COVID-19 virus RNA immediately takes control of the human cell's protein synthesis system and starts making its own proteins and other components needed for making new COVID-19 virus particles.

One of the COVID-19 proteins is the spike protein (S protein). The S protein, produced inside our cells, will soon be detected by our immune system. The immune system therefore starts making antibodies against the S proteins. It also makes antibodies against some of the other COVID-19 virus proteins. As we've seen in the preceding chapters, antibodies against the S protein are important because they can block the entry of the COVID-19 virus into our cells. In most of the clinical trials of COVID-19 vaccine candidates, the production of neutralizing antibodies against the COVID-19 S protein is used as a measure for the effectiveness of the vaccine.

THE IDEA BEHIND THE MRNA COVID-19 VACCINES

As we've seen in the preceding chapters, some of the most effective vaccines are vaccines that multiply inside human cells and start making copies of the virus or virus proteins that the vaccine is intended to protect against.

Scientists hope that the complicated and lengthy process of making a live attenuated virus, or a viral vector vaccine, can be avoided by directly injecting the mRNA coding for the protein of interest into human cells. The idea behind this is that the result of vaccination with viral vector vaccines or live attenuated vaccines is the production of the virus mRNA inside our cells. It is therefore an obvious thought that it would be much easier to make the mRNA and inject it rather than first making a live attenuated vaccine or a virus vector vaccine.

The main technical advantage of this technology is that mRNA can be synthesized through enzymatic or chemical methods.

There is thus no need for any host cell or cell cultures. This makes it faster to develop a new type of mRNA vaccine. The manufacturing of the mRNA itself is easy to scale up, although the encapsulation of the mRNA into nano lipid particles might be a bottleneck according to some sources. Making many millions or billions of an mRNA vaccine will meet some of the same challenges as other vaccine types. The mRNA needs to be filled into a vial or syringe, and there may be a temporary shortage of vials, syringes, and needles.

SELECTING THE RIGHT MRNA

There are some challenges in making an mRNA vaccine against the COVID-19 proteins. First, scientists must choose the "right" piece of mRNA. This does not need to be a complicated task, as the gene sequence for the COVID-19 virus and for any of its proteins, including the spike protein, has been known since early this year (2020).

The scientists must, however, decide which protein and which part of the protein the vaccine must target. Often, the S protein or a part of it, for example the Receptor-Binding Domain (RBD), is used as a target.

The mRNA to be used as a vaccine does not need to look exactly the same as the mRNA produced in our cells infected by the COVID-19 virus. It must, however, be able to initiate and direct the synthesis of the COVID-19 protein in the same way as the COVID-19 virus mRNA would. The scientists can modify the mRNA to be used as a vaccine in various ways to create a more effective and long-lasting immune response.

GETTING THE MRNA INTO HUMAN CELLS

Next, the scientists must find a way to get the mRNA into human cells. The mRNA is a large and fragile molecule, which cannot by itself get into human cells. It needs to be wrapped in a lipid particle to ease its entry into our cells and to protect it against degradation. The commonly used approach is to encapsulate the mRNA in a nanoparticle (a very small particle; see below) consisting of lipids. These particles are called lipid nanoparticles (LNPs). Three of the mRNA vaccines that were in clinical trials (as of June 24) are LNP mRNA vaccines. The fourth mRNA vaccine from CureVac may also be using this technology, but CureVac does have access to another technology for getting mRNA into the cells (see below).

Our cells have a lipid membrane, and it is relatively easy for a lipid nanoparticle to enter human cells. The LNP works as a shuttle that delivers the RNA inside the cells.

By the way, the fancy name "nanoparticles," which is also used for some products like nanoparticle paint, just means that the particles are less than one millionth of one meter in diameter. The name thus refers to the size of the particles.

Whereas it's possible to make large amounts of mRNA within a short time, one bottleneck in the manufacturing of mRNA vaccines may be the encapsulation of the RNA within lipid nanoparticles. As mentioned above, another bottleneck may be the shortage of the vials, syringes, and needles that are needed to deliver the vaccine in small vials (or prefilled single-use syringes) to be used for the vaccination.

Whereas no vaccine based on RNA technology has been brought to the market yet, there have been several trials of mRNA vaccine candidates in humans. It is not clear why none of these candidates did not move forward to Phase 3 studies and commercial manufacturing. One reason why might be because the mRNA vaccine candidates developed so far have not been effective enough, or because they may have had too many or too severe adverse effects. Another possibility is that the companies have not been able to raise enough capital to fund the expensive late-stage development of such vaccines. Phase 3 clinical trials are very expensive, and strong proof of safety and effectiveness would be needed to persuade a big pharma company or an investor to commit to the further development of a new vaccine type.

THE FOUR MRNA COVID-19 VACCINES IN CLINICAL TRIALS

As mentioned above, there were four COVID-19 vaccine candidates based on the mRNA technology in clinical trials as of June 24. Below we'll explore each of the four mRNA COVID-19 vaccine lead candidates.

THE MRNA-1273 COVID-19 VACCINE FROM MODERNA

The COVID-19 vaccine candidate made by Moderna and being tested in humans is named mRNA-1273. This mRNA codes for the COVID-19 spike protein. As mentioned, the mRNA has been encapsulated in lipid nanoparticles.

THE PHASE 1 CLINICAL TRIAL

The Phase 1 clinical trial of this vaccine began on February 25, 2020. It is an open study, which means that the doctors, the test subjects, and any other person involved in the trial know whether a test subject gets the COVID-19 S protein vaccine or a placebo. They will also know which dose a test subject gets. Moderna will test five different doses: 10, 25, 50, 100, and 250 micrograms to define the optimal dose in subsequent trials.

The study has been designed as a two-dose study. This means that the test subjects will receive first a prime dose, and then after one month (28 days), a second booster dose. This may have been decided to ensure an effective immune response.

The 155 participants have been divided into 13 groups (called arms in clinical trials). This is partly due to the five dose levels to be tested, but also due to the division of the participants into three age groups. The 155 participants have thus been divided into three age groups: 18–55, 56–70, and 71–99 years old. Inclusion of the latter group is interesting, as this is the group that is most vulnerable to COVID-19 infections and most likely to get the severe COVID-19 disease. Most patients who have died from the COVID-19 infection have been over 70 years old—and the highest death rate was seen in people over 80 years old.

The investigators will observe the test subjects for local adverse events (redness, heat, swelling, or pain at the injection site) and for systemic adverse events such as fever. They will also evaluate the effectiveness of the vaccine by its ability to produce IgG antibodies in the vaccinated subjects.

According to the published clinical trial protocol, measurement of neutralizing antibodies against the COVID-19 virus does not seem to have been included in the Phase 1 trial. However, in a press release, Moderna reported that they have measured neutralizing antibodies in eight participants. They stated that vaccination with the mRNA-1273 resulted in the development of neutralizing antibodies in the first eight participants given 25 micrograms or 100 micrograms of the mRNA-1273 vaccine. They also stated that the vaccine was generally safe and well tolerated.

THE PHASE 2 CLINICAL TRIAL

On May 13, 2020, Moderna filed an application for a Phase 2 clinical trial of their mRNA-1273 vaccine. In the Phase 2 trial, Moderna plan to enroll 600 participants older than 18 years old. The doses to be tested have been narrowed down to 50 micrograms and 100 micrograms, whereas they ranged from 25 micrograms to 250 micrograms in the Phase 1 trial (see above).

In contrast to the Phase 1 trial, the Phase 2 trial will be blinded (see Chapter 4). In addition, Moderna will also measure neutralizing antibodies against the COVID-19 virus.

LARGE-SCALE MANUFACTURING OF THE MRNA-1273 VACCINE

The Biomedical Advanced Research and Development Authority (BARDA) has awarded Moderna up to $483 million to accelerate development of mRNA-1273 to enable large-scale production in 2020 for pandemic response. In addition, Moderna made an alliance with the large-scale contract manufacturing organization Lonza. Moderna's goal is to be able to manufacture up to one billion doses of the m1273 COVID-19 vaccine per year.

Moderna stated that it may take 12 to 18 months before their m1273 vaccine becomes commercially available. However, they envisage that the vaccine could become available under emergency authorization to some people, including healthcare workers, as early as in the fall of 2020.

THE BIONTECH MRNA VACCINE CANDIDATES

BioNTech is a German company that, like Moderna, has worked with mRNA vaccine technology for several years. They have focused on developing vaccine candidates to stimulate cancer patients' immune response against cancer. Several of their cancer immunotherapy vaccines have entered clinical trial testing.

In the past, they've made several other vaccines against viruses. One of these was a vaccine candidate against the Zika virus. They showed in a study with rhesus monkeys that a single vaccine dose of 50 micrograms protected the monkeys from becoming ill when exposed to the Zika virus. There seems to be no published similar study of their COVID-19 mRNA vaccine candidates. However, in a presentation from April 23, 2020, they stated that they have demonstrated a high efficacy of their mRNA COVID-19 vaccine candidates (see below).

BioNTech have developed several mRNA COVID-19 vaccine candidates. Their lead candidate is called BNT162. From the US clinical trial (see below) and from one of their presentations, it appears that the four candidates to be tested are named 162a1, 162b1, 162b2, and 162c1. In a presentation from April 23, 2020, (please see "References" at the end of the chapter), BioNTech partly revealed the chemical nature of the four mRNA vaccine candidates.

Two of them are nucleoside-modified mRNA vaccines. This just implies that one or more of the four building blocks in RNA, called nucleotides, have been exchanged with a modified nucleotide. The four building blocks are A (adenine), C (cytosine), G (guanine), and U (uracil). BioNTech states that nucleoside-modified mRNA vaccines can produce a very strong antibody response.

The third type is called a uridine-modified RNA vaccine, and the fourth type is a self-amplifying RNA vaccine. As the name implies, the latter type of mRNA vaccine can replicate itself inside the cells and hence may induce a strong and long-lasting immune response—like a live attenuated vaccine (see Chapter 6).

All four mRNA vaccines have been encapsulated in lipid nanoparticles. Some of them target larger parts of the COVID-19 S protein, whereas one (or more) targets the Receptor-Binding Domain (RBD) of the S protein.

BIONTECH HAVE PARTNERED WITH BOTH A CHINESE AND A US PHARMA COMPANY

BioNTech have teamed up with two pharmaceutical companies. On March 16, 2020, they agreed with the Shanghai-based Chinese company Fosun Pharma to co-develop their lead COVID-19 mRNA vaccine candidate. They plan, among other things, to conduct clinical trials of their lead candidate BN162. Fosun Pharma will pay $135 million in upfront and milestone payments.

On March 17, 2020, BioNTech also made an agreement with the US big pharma company, Pfizer, about the co-development of their lead candidate: the BN162 mRNA vaccine. Later, the agreement was expanded to include several COVID-19 mRNA vaccine candidates (see below). Pfizer have agreed to pay BioNTech an upfront payment of $185 million. BioNTech and Pfizer strive to have millions of doses ready by the end of 2020.

THE BIONTECH CLINICAL TRIALS

BioNTech have applied for permission to conduct clinical trials with their COVID-19 mRNA vaccine candidates in both the EU and the US. In collaboration with their Chinese partner, Fosun Pharma, they will also apply to begin clinical trials in China. The application has not been filed yet (June 19, 2020). The title of the trial application is "A Phase 1/2, Placebo-Controlled, Randomized, Observer-Blind, Dose-Finding Study to Describe the Safety, Tolerability, Immunogenicity, And Potential Efficacy of Sars-Cov-2 RNA Vaccine Candidates Against Covid-19 In Healthy Adults."

In the US trial, BioNTech plan to enroll 7,600 participants. The test subjects will receive one or two doses, and up to three dose levels will be tested. The participants will be divided into three age groups: 18–55, 65–85, and 18–85 years old.

The investigators will evaluate four different COVID-19 mRNA vaccine candidates named 162a1, 162b1, 162b2, and 162c1. The four candidates target larger or smaller parts of the S protein. The mRNAs to be used in all four candidates seem to have been modified in various ways (see above).

The participants will be observed for any adverse events and changes in blood chemistry. To evaluate the effectiveness of the vaccines, the investigators will measure neutralizing antibodies in blood specimens at appropriate intervals.

The EU clinical trial application does not contain as many details as the US application, but the US application gives us a clear picture of the clinical trials that BioNTech is going to conduct.

FIRST RESULTS FROM THE BIONTECH CLINICAL TRIALS

When I was preparing the book for printing (July 2), the first results from the clinical trial conducted in collaboration with Pfizer were reported. The mRNA vaccine used was the nucleoside modified BNT162b1.

The results from the first 45 participants, of which 36 received the vaccine and nine a placebo, showed that pain at the injection site was the most frequent adverse event. All local reactions were mild or moderate in severity, except for one test subject, who had severe pain after being vaccinated with the highest dose (100 micrograms).

Several test subjects also had fever, fatigue, headache, chills, and muscle or joint pain. These adverse events were dose-dependent. They generally peaked at Day 2 after the vaccination and had disappeared by Day 7. Transient decrease in the white blood cells were also seen in some participants.

The vaccinated subjects produced neutralizing antibodies against the Receptor-Binding Domain of the COVID-19 S protein. The level produced was higher than the level found in sera from patients that have had a natural COVID-19 virus infection (convalescence sera). The level of neutralizing antibodies increased with increasing dose and was significantly higher after a second dose.

The results indicate that it may be possible to find a well-tolerated dose that produces good immunity after two doses.

THE LNP-NCOVSARNA VACCINE FROM IMPERIAL COLLEGE LONDON

Imperial College London is a public research university in London, England. Their RNA COVID-19 vaccine is based on self-amplifying messenger RNA (mRNA). This means that the mRNA starts replicating itself when it has entered our cells. Therefore, according to Imperial College London, only very small amounts of mRNA should be needed to generate a strong immune response. The institute claims that they can manufacture one million doses in a reaction vessel with a volume of only one liter.

As with the other RNA vaccines that we have learned about, the LNP-nCoVsaRNA has been encapsulated in lipid nanoparticles to protect the mRNA against degradation and to ease the uptake in our cells.

The Phase 1 study will enroll about 300 participants ranging from 18 to 75 years old. The first doses will be administered in the younger participants (18–45 years old). The investigators will test three doses: 0.1 microgram, 0.3 microgram, and 1.0 microgram.

THE CUREVAC MRNA VACCINE

CureVac is a German company that has extensive experience in working with mRNA vaccines. They received permission to start clinical trials with their mRNA vaccine that targets the COVID-19 S protein. CureVac has access to two technologies for delivering mRNA vaccines into the cells. One is based on the LNP technology that is also used by some of the other companies to develop mRNA vaccines. The other, the CureVac Carrier Molecule (CVCM), has been developed by CureVac. The clinical trial protocol had not been published when I finished editing the book on June 24, 2020, so I cannot provide any further details.

KEY TAKEAWAYS

Vaccines based on mRNA are a new promising technology. The result of vaccination with some other types of vaccines against the COVID-19 virus is that our cells start producing the mRNA coding for the COVID-19 proteins. The idea behind mRNA vaccines is to bypass the complex process of making vaccines such as viral vector vaccines and live attenuated vaccines in cell cultures. Instead, the mRNA coding for the S protein is injected directly into the human body.

Although several mRNA vaccine candidates have been tested in clinical trials, no mRNA vaccine candidate has been licensed yet. Most of them have only been tested in a small number of test subjects. It is therefore unknown whether they are safe and effective.

It also remains to be proven whether mRNA vaccines can be produced in millions or billions of doses. The scale-up of the mRNA synthesis should not be a big challenge, but the encapsulation of the mRNA in lipid nanoparticles might according to some sources become a bottleneck. Temporary shortage of vials, syringes, and needles may also hinder the production of one billion doses within a short time.

Four of the 16 COVID-19 vaccine candidates are based on the mRNA technology. They have been developed by the US company Moderna, the German company BioNTech, the UK research institute Imperial College London, and the German company CureVac. We know only little about the Moderna and the CureVac vaccines. BioNTech has developed four different mRNA vaccines, which are all going to be tested in clinical trials. One is a self-replicating mRNA vaccine. The vaccine from Imperial College London is also a self-replicating vaccine. Self-replicating mRNA vaccines should at least in theory produce a stronger immune response than other mRNA vaccines.

When I finished editing this book (June 24), Moderna, BioNTech, and Imperial College London had initiated clinical trials with their vaccine candidates. CureVac had not yet published their clinical trial protocol.

Both Moderna and BioNTech have teamed up with strong partners capable of large-scale manufacturing. They have also received strong financial support. CureVac has received financial support from the German Government, which has bought stocks in the company for €300 million.

Moderna has released initial results via press releases. When I prepared the book for printing (July 2), BioNTech published initial results from the clinical trial conducted in collaboration with Pfizer. The results indicate that it may be possible to find a well-tolerated dose that produces good immunity after two doses.

The positive results from two of the companies give us hope that it may be possible to deliver many doses of COVID-19 mRNA vaccines under emergency-use authorization in 2020.

REFERENCES

Cross, R. 2020. "Will the coronavirus help mRNA and DNA vaccines prove their worth?". Chemical & Engineering News, Last Modified April 14, accessed July 4. https://cen.acs.org/pharmaceuticals/vaccines/coronavirus-help-mRNA-DNA-vaccines/98/i14.

Gomez-Aguado, I., J. Rodriguez-Castejon, M. Vicente-Pascual, A. Rodriguez-Gascon, M. A. Solinis, and A. Del Pozo-Rodriguez. 2020. "Nanomedicines to Deliver mRNA: State of the Art and Future Perspectives." *Nanomaterials (Basel)* 10 (2).

Liu, M. A. 2019. "A Comparison of Plasmid DNA and mRNA as Vaccine Technologies." *Vaccines (Basel)* 7 (2).

Moderna. 2020. "Moderna Announces Positive Interim Phase 1 Data for its mRNA Vaccine (mRNA-1273) Against Novel Coronavirus." [Press Release], Last Modified May 18, accessed July 4. https://investors.modernatx.com/news-releases/news-release-details/moderna-announces-positive-interim-phase-1-data-its-mrna-vaccine.

Muligan, MJ; Lyke, KE; Kitchin, N. et al. 2020. "Phase 1/2 Study to Describe the Safety and Immunogenicity of a COVID-19 RNA Vaccine Candidate (BNT162b1) in Adults 18 to 55 Years of Age: Interim Report." MedRxiv, accessed July 4. https://www.medrxiv.org/content/10.1101/2020.06.30.20142570v1.

Pardi, N., M. J. Hogan, R. S. Pelc, H. Muramatsu, H. Andersen, C. R. DeMaso, K. A. Dowd, L. L. Sutherland, R. M. Scearce, R. Parks, W. Wagner, A. Granados, J. Greenhouse, M. Walker, E. Willis, J. S. Yu, C. E. McGee, G. D. Sempowski, B. L. Mui, Y. K. Tam, Y. J. Huang, D. Vanlandingham, V. M. Holmes, H. Balachandran, S. Sahu, M. Lifton, S. Higgs, S. E. Hensley, T. D. Madden, M. J. Hope, K. Kariko, S. Santra, B. S. Graham, M. G. Lewis, T. C. Pierson, B. F. Haynes, and D. Weissman. 2017. "Zika virus protection by a single low-dose nucleoside-modified mRNA vaccination." *Nature* 543 (7644):248-251.

Reichmuth, A. M., M. A. Oberli, A. Jaklenec, R. Langer, and D. Blankschtein. 2016. "mRNA vaccine delivery using lipid nanoparticles." *Ther Deliv* 7 (5):319-34.

Wang, F., R. M. Kream, and G. B. Stefano. 2020. "An Evidence Based Perspective on mRNA-SARS-CoV-2 Vaccine Development." *Med Sci Monit* 26:e924700..

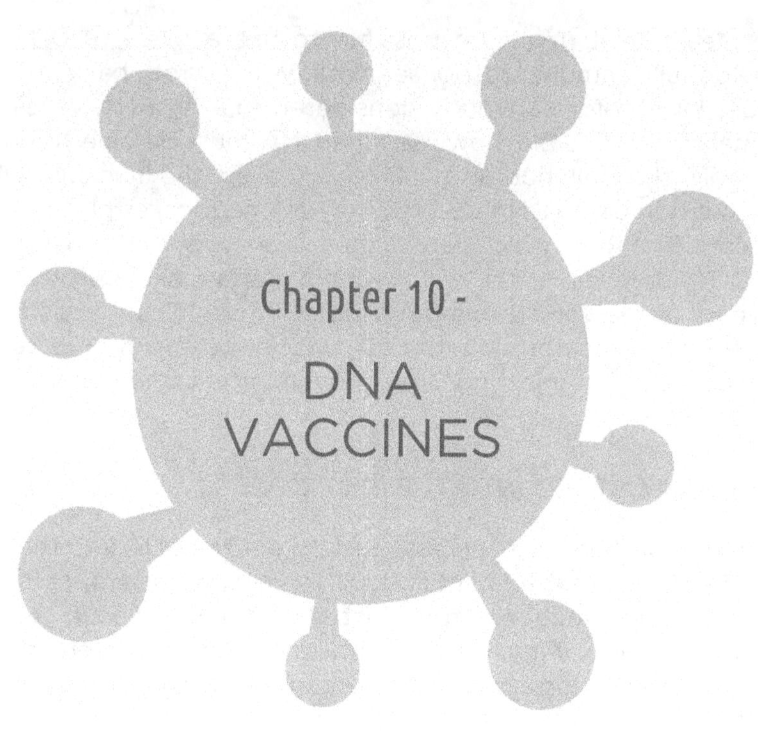

Chapter 10 -
DNA VACCINES

As you may recall from Chapter 6 and Chapter 9, our genes consist of DNA. This DNA contains the information needed to make the proteins that make up our cells. All bacteria and many viruses also use DNA as the code for their proteins, whereas some viruses use RNA as the code.

USE OF DNA AS A VACCINE

The idea that it might be possible to use a piece of DNA to develop an immune response already occurred back in the 1950s—long before anybody considered making RNA vaccines. To make this possible, however, the DNA must be able to enter not only the cell but also its core (called the nucleus). The transcription of the DNA code to the RNA code takes place in the cell core. The RNA, which carries the same genetic information as the DNA, then leaves the cell core and starts making proteins in the part of the cell surrounding the cell core. This is called the cytosol. The breakthrough for DNA vaccines came in 1990, when it was shown that injecting DNA into a muscle could generate an immune response.

THE DNA MUST GET INTO THE CELL CORE

It turned out that it isn't an easy task to get the DNA into the cell core. In the early experiments with DNA vaccines, scientists found that only a tiny fraction of the injected DNA succeeded in getting into the cell core. Initially, the scientists were mainly interested in the DNA technology to try to cure genetic diseases by gene therapy. The general idea was to attempt to build in the part of the DNA that the patient was missing. It was also attempted to use gene therapy for the treatment of cancers.

FROM GENE THERAPY TO VACCINES

Among other things, due to the technical challenges met with gene therapy, many scientists started exploring the use of DNA as vaccines against infectious diseases. To be effective as gene therapy, a long-lasting or permanent production of the protein that the patient with the genetic disease is missing is needed. In contrast, a vaccine DNA only needs to be effective for a short time to create a strong antibody and T-cell response. In recent years, there has been an increased understanding of how DNA vaccines work, and the steps needed for a DNA vaccine to create an immune response have been improved.

A DNA VACCINE IS A SMALL RING OF DNA FROM A BACTERIUM

A DNA vaccine consists of a small ring of DNA. This ring stems from a bacterium, and DNA vaccines are actually manufactured in bacteria. The small DNA rings are called plasmids, a scientific term that we'll also use. Within a bacterium, the plasmids exist outside the bacterium's own DNA (the chromosomal DNA), and they can replicate independently of the bacterial DNA. Bacteria are easy to grow in labs and in large-scale production units. The plasmids are very stable and easy to purify. DNA vaccines can be stored at ambient temperatures for a long time, which also makes them ideal for use in countries with hot climates. All these factors make DNA vaccines an attractive technology.

INSERTING COVID-19 GENES INTO THE DNA VACCINE

When scientists want to make a DNA vaccine against a part of the COVID-19 virus, they insert the gene for the protein that they want to make into the plasmid DNA. The plasmid DNA is then developed in the bacteria and purified for use in animals or humans. As an example, the gene coding for the COVID-19 spike protein (S protein) may be inserted into a plasmid. Together with the gene of interest, here the gene coding for the S protein, other genes are often also built into the plasmid to enhance the transcription of the DNA to RNA or to enhance the immune response.

HOW THE DNA VACCINE GETS INTO THE CELL AND CELL CORE

One of the biggest challenges with a DNA vaccine is how to get it into the human cells and into the core of the cells. Various methods for this have been developed. A DNA vaccine can simply be injected into a muscle (the same way as used for many other vaccines), but this may not lead to an effective immune response.

Other more effective methods to get DNA vaccines into the cells have been developed. In one method, the vaccine is injected into the skin. The uptake of the vaccine into the cells is then subsequently enhanced by applying an electric field over the injection site. This method or process is called electroporation. Electroporation works by making it easier for the DNA to enter the cells through the cell membranes. One of the DNA COVID-19 vaccines currently in clinical trial (June 24, 2020)—the INO-4800 vaccine (see below)—is based on this method for getting the DNA into the cells.

With another method, the DNA vaccine is coated on gold particles that are then at a high pressure injected into the cells by using a "gene gun." Today, this technology is mainly used in plant biotechnology. We won't explore this technology any further.

HOW THE DNA ENTERS THE CELL CORE

When the DNA has entered the cell, it must also be taken up in the cell core. For this to happen, it must be able to penetrate the cell core membrane. Essentially, the DNA plasmid has to make it to the cell core by using the cell's own systems to transport molecules. After a DNA vaccine has entered the cell, it binds to a number of the cell's own proteins. Together, they move inside some tiny tubes (called microtubules) until they reach the cell core.

When the DNA vaccine has entered the cell core, it starts behaving like our own DNA. This means that it will start making the RNA that codes for the COVID-19 protein. The RNA then leaves the cell core and starts making the COVID-19 proteins in the fluid (cytoplasm) surrounding the cell core.

The COVID-19 virus proteins made by the RNA will be recognized by the immune system as being foreign proteins, and the body will start producing an immune response against the COVID-19 protein.

DNA VACCINES AGAINST ANIMAL INFECTIOUS DISEASES

There are no licensed DNA vaccines for use against human infections on the market. However, three DNA vaccines against infectious diseases have been licensed for use in animals. Two of them are used to prevent certain diseases affecting fish. The third vaccine was licensed for preventing the West Nile virus (WNV) infection in horses. It turned out to also be effective for preventing the WNV infection in birds, for example the condor.

It was previously thought that DNA vaccines would not be able to generate a strong immune response in larger animals. However, the existence of a licensed DNA vaccine for use in horses indicates that it should also be possible to develop a vaccine against the COVID-19 disease to be used in humans.

DNA VACCINES AGAINST OTHER CORONAVIRUSES

Before the COVID-19 pandemic, DNA vaccine candidates against the two other known severe coronaviruses causing the diseases SARS and MERS had been developed and tested in animal studies and clinical trials. Clinical trials of SARS DNA vaccines are particularly interesting, because both the SARS and the COVID-19 virus use the same way of entering the human cells, namely via the ACE2 receptor. They both attach to the ACE2 receptor via the S protein Receptor-Binding Domain (RBD). In contrast, the MERS virus uses another receptor to enter human cells.

THE SARS DNA VACCINE CLINICAL TRIAL

In a clinical trial conducted in 2008, a SARS DNA vaccine candidate was tested in 10 healthy adults in a Phase 1 clinical trial. Each test subject received three doses of the DNA vaccine against SARS. Nine of the 10 test subjects completed all three doses. The vaccine was administered using the Biojector 2000® Needle-Free Injection Management System™. This means that no electroporation was used to enhance the uptake of the vaccine in the muscle.

All nine subjects that received all three doses developed neutralizing antibodies. Two of the test subjects produced only low levels of neutralizing antibodies, but five produced high levels. The level of neutralizing antibodies peaked after 12 weeks, but neutralizing antibodies were still present in blood specimens from most vaccinated subjects after 32 weeks.

Some of the participants experienced mild local adverse events, but none of them had any severe adverse event. The SARS DNA vaccine was thus well tolerated.

The results from this trial back in 2008 indicate that it is possible to develop a safe DNA vaccine against the SARS coronavirus that may protect the vaccinated subject for half a year or more. Since then, the technology for injection of DNA vaccines has been improved. Today, electroporation is used to enhance the uptake of the DNA vaccine. This may improve the effectiveness of the vaccine.

THE INOVIO MERS DNA VACCINE CLINICAL TRIAL

Inovio previously developed a DNA vaccine against the MERS disease: the INO-4700. The DNA vaccine contained the gene for the MERS S protein, which is almost identical to the COVID-19 S protein.

Under the name GLS-5300, the INO-4700 DNA vaccine has been tested in a Phase 1 clinical trial enrolling 75 healthy adults. The test subjects were divided into three groups that received 0.67 milligrams, two milligrams, or six milligrams of the vaccine. All test subjects got three doses at week 0 (the start of the study), week 4, and week 12. 66 of the participants completed the vaccine schedule and received all three doses.

The participants developed both antibodies and a T-cell response to the MERS S protein. Already after the second vaccination, most participants had developed IgG antibodies against the MERS S protein. The antibody level remained high after 60 weeks. The participants first started producing neutralizing antibodies after the third vaccination. After 60 weeks, the level of neutralizing antibodies had decreased, and only two of the 66 participants had significant levels of neutralizing antibodies.

The investigators concluded that the MERS DNA vaccine was well tolerated, and that more than 85% of the participants developed an immune response already after two vaccinations.

As we saw above, the IgG antibody response lasted more than one year, but the level of neutralizing antibodies first rose after the third vaccination and had decreased significantly after 60 weeks. However, this does not necessarily mean that the MERS DNA vaccine would not be effective for a longer time. It is likely that memory B and T cells may have been formed after three doses of vaccination, and that the level of IgG antibodies remained high after one year.

In conclusion, the results from the clinical trial of the INO-4700 MERS DNA vaccine, which in many ways is similar to the COVID-19 INO-4800 DNA vaccine, indicate that it may be possible to make a safe and effective DNA vaccine against the COVID-19 disease.

TESTING A COVID-19 DNA VACCINE IN RHESUS MONKEYS

No results from testing a COVID-19 DNA vaccine in humans have been published yet. However, six DNA vaccines protecting against the COVID-19 virus have been developed by a group of scientists and tested in rhesus monkeys. All six vaccines targeted the S protein or parts hereof. One vaccine candidate targeted the full-length S protein, and one candidate targeted the S protein receptor-binding domain, whereas the other four candidates targeted various other forms of the S protein.

The monkeys were divided into seven groups—one for each of the six vaccine candidates and one control group. There were four or five animals in each of the vaccine groups and 10 animals in the control group.

Each monkey received two injections of the vaccine at week 0 and week 3. After five weeks (two weeks after the last vaccination), all animals vaccinated with one of the six vaccine candidates, the full-length S protein, had developed neutralizing antibodies.

After six weeks (three weeks after the second vaccination), the scientists exposed the animals to a high dose (12 million virus particles) of the COVID-19 virus. They gave the animals COVID-19 in their noses and windpipes. They then examined the noses and lungs for the presence of the COVID-19 virus. The monkeys had only mild symptoms. No COVID-19 virus RNA was found in blood specimens. Compared to the control animals, the vaccinated animals had 1,000 times fewer COVID-19 virus particles in the secretion from the nose, and 5,000 times fewer COVID-19 virus particles in the fluid aspirated from the lungs.

The scientists concluded that a vaccine with DNA coding for the full-length COVID-19 S protein gave good protection against COVID-19 lung infections. In addition, the level of COVID-19 neutralizing antibodies seemed to predict how effective the vaccine is when the animals are infected with the COVID-19 virus.

The results indicate that it may be possible to develop a COVID-19 DNA vaccine, and that the level of neutralizing antibodies against the S protein may be used to assess whether a given person would be protected against a COVID-19 infection.

THE INOVIO DNA VACCINE AGAINST COVID-19

The US company Inovio has developed a DNA vaccine candidate against COVID-19 virus. The DNA vaccine contains the gene for the COVID-19 virus S protein. It has been given the name INO-4800.

TESTING THE INO-4800 IN ANIMALS

The INO-4800 has been tested in mice and guinea pigs, but not yet in monkeys (June 24, 2020). Here, we'll only look at the results from the guinea pigs. Each guinea pig received three doses of 100 Qg of the vaccine. The production of antibodies was measured by two different methods. With both methods, the guinea pigs produced high levels of neutralizing antibodies (titers greater than 320).

THE INO-4800 CLINICAL TRIAL

The investigators will test the INO-4800 DNA vaccine in a Phase 1 clinical trial with 120 participants. They have divided the test subjects into three groups that will receive 0.5, 1.0, or 2.0 milligrams of the vaccine. The vaccine will be injected directly into the skin—unlike most other vaccines, which are administered under the skin or into a muscle. Injection into the skin is an effective way to create a strong immune response.

The trial is an open study, so both the investigators and the participants will know which dose a given test subject gets. There is no control group. The test subject in all three dose groups will receive two doses: one at their first visit (day 0) and one after four weeks. The uptake of the DNA vaccine into the cells will be enhanced by electroporation, using Inovio's electroporation device CELLECTRA® 2000. The purpose of the electroporation is to open up the pores in the cells so that it's easier for the DNA to enter the cells.

The investigators will assess the safety of the DNA vaccine and its effectiveness. They will also observe the participants for any adverse reactions, as well as assess the vaccine's effectiveness by measuring IgG antibodies against the S protein and by measuring interferon gamma (INF-γ). INF-γ is secreted by the T cell and can be used as a measure for T-cell activation. The study will be completed in July 2021, but some results may be published earlier.

THE GENEXINE GX-19 DNA VACCINE

Genexine is a Korean biotech company. They have developed a DNA vaccine, the GX-19 vaccine, against the COVID-19 virus. After vaccination, it produces the COVID-19 S protein inside our cells.

The investigators have begun a Phase 1/2 study of the Genexine GX-19 vaccine. They plan to enroll 190 participants, who will be divided into three groups. One group will receive saline as a placebo. The two other groups will receive the DNA vaccine in two different doses. All three groups will receive two injections with a four-week interval between each dose.

Apparently, no information about the use of electroporation or other means for easing the uptake of the COVID-19 DNA vaccine in the cells has been published. However, the company has previously developed another DNA vaccine against HPV cervical cancer. For this vaccine, they used electroporation to enhance the uptake. The HPV DNA vaccine successfully completed Phase 2 clinical trial.

The investigators will monitor the participants for any adverse events. To assess the effectiveness of the vaccine, they will measure IgG and neutralizing antibodies. They will also measure the T cells' response to the COVID-19 S protein. The study had just begun when I finished editing this book. No results are available yet.

KEY TAKEAWAYS

Experiments with DNA vaccines started back in the 1950s. The breakthrough came when it was shown that injection of DNA into a muscle could generate an immune response.

Initially, the main interest in DNA vaccines was to attempt to cure genetic diseases by replacing the gene that the patient was missing. Scientists also attempted to treat cancer with DNA vaccines.

Among other things, due to the technical challenges met by gene therapy and treatment of cancers with DNA vaccines, the interest in using DNA vaccines to protect against infectious disease increased.

One challenge of DNA vaccines is that the vaccine must not only enter the cell—it must also enter the cell core. The uptake of the DNA vaccine may be enhanced by use of electroporation, which opens the pores in the cells.

No DNA vaccine to be used in humans has yet been approved, but there exist three licensed vaccines for animal infectious diseases, one of which is for protecting horses against the West Nile virus infection. This indicates that it should also be possible to develop DNA vaccines against human infectious diseases.

Scientists have developed and tested DNA vaccines against the two dangerous coronaviruses that cause the MERS and SARS diseases. Both types of vaccines have been tested in animal studies and clinical trials. The results of the clinical trials indicate that it should be possible to develop a safe and effective DNA vaccine against the COVID-19 disease.

COVID-19 vaccine candidates have shown promising results in animal studies. Six candidates were tested in rhesus monkeys. The scientists found that one of the six DNA vaccines targeting the full-length S protein protected the monkeys against getting a severe COVID-19 disease. They also found that the level of neutralizing antibodies predicted the ability of the vaccine to protect against the COVID-19 disease.

When I finished editing this chapter (June 24, 2020), there were two DNA COVID-19 vaccines in clinical trial.

One vaccine was the INO-4800 from Inovio. Inovio previously made an effective MERS DNA vaccine candidate. This increases the likelihood that their COVID-19 DNA vaccine candidate will be safe and effective.

The other vaccine GX-19 was from the Korean company Genexine. They have previously developed an HPV cervical cancer vaccine that has been tested in a Phase 2 clinical trial. This also increases the likelihood that their COVID-19 DNA vaccine will be effective and safe.

Altogether, the two DNA vaccines in clinical trials should have a good chance of success. They are both made by companies who are experienced in DNA vaccines and who have made other DNA vaccines before. DNA vaccines against SARS and MERS have successfully been made before.

REFERENCES

Bolhassani, A., and S. R. Yazdi. 2009. "DNA immunization as an efficient strategy for vaccination." *Avicenna J Med Biotechnol* 1 (2):71-88.

Hobernik, D; Bros, M. 2018. "DNA Vaccines—How Far From Clinical Use?" *Int J Mol Sci* 19 (11).

Inovio. 2020. "INOVIO Announces Positive Interim Phase 1 Data For INO-4800 Vaccine for COVID-19." [Press Release]. Inovio, accessed July 4. http://s23.q4cdn.com/479936946/files/doc_news/INOVIO-Announces-Positive-Interim-Phase-1-Data-For-INO-4800-Vaccine-for-COVID-19-2020.pdf.

Martin, J. E., M. K. Louder, L. A. Holman, I. J. Gordon, M. E. Enama, B. D. Larkin, C. A. Andrews, L. Vogel, R. A. Koup, M. Roederer, R. T. Bailer, P. L. Gomez, M. Nason, J. R. Mascola, G. J. Nabel, B. S. Graham, and V. R. C. Study Team. 2008. "A SARS DNA vaccine induces neutralizing antibody and cellular immune responses in healthy adults in a Phase I clinical trial." *Vaccine* 26 (50):6338-43.

Modjarrad, K., C. C. Roberts, K. T. Mills, A. R. Castellano, K. Paolino, K. Muthumani, E. L. Reuschel, M. L. Robb, T. Racine, M. D. Oh, C. Lamarre, F. I. Zaidi, J. Boyer, S. B. Kudchodkar, M. Jeong, J. M. Darden, Y. K. Park, P. T. Scott, C. Remigio, A. P. Parikh, M. C. Wise, A. Patel, E. K. Duperret, K. Y. Kim, H. Choi, S. White, M. Bagarazzi, J. M. May, D. Kane, H. Lee, G. Kobinger, N. L. Michael, D. B. Weiner, S. J. Thomas, and J. N. Maslow. 2019. "Safety and immunogenicity of an anti-Middle East respiratory syndrome coronavirus DNA vaccine: a phase 1, open-label, single-arm, dose-escalation trial." *Lancet Infect Dis* 19 (9):1013-1022.

Moreno, S., Timon. 2004. "DNA vaccination: an immunological perspective." *Immunolia* 23 (1):41.

Muthumani, K., D. Falzarano, E. L. Reuschel, C. Tingey, S. Flingai, D. O. Villarreal, M. Wise, A. Patel, A. Izmirly, A. Aljuaid, A. M. Seliga, G. Soule, M. Morrow, K. A. Kraynyak, A. S. Khan, D. P. Scott, F. Feldmann, R. LaCasse, K. Meade-White, A. Okumura, K. E. Ugen, N. Y. Sardesai, J. J. Kim, G. Kobinger, H. Feldmann, and D. B. Weiner. 2015. "A synthetic consensus anti-spike protein DNA vaccine induces protective immunity against Middle East respiratory syndrome coronavirus in nonhuman primates." *Sci Transl Med* 7 (301):301ra132.

Rosa, DS; de Souzxa Apostolico; J; Boscardin, SB. 2015. "DNA Vaccines: How Much Have We Accomplished In The Last 25 Years?" *Journal of Vaccines & Vaccination* 6 (3).

Smith, T. R. F., A. Patel, S. Ramos, D. Elwood, X. Zhu, J. Yan, E. N. Gary, S. N. Walker, K. Schultheis, M. Purwar, Z. Xu, J. Walters, P. Bhojnagarwala, M. Yang, N. Chokkalingam, P. Pezzoli, E. Parzych, E. L. Reuschel, A. Doan, N. Tursi, M. Vasquez, J. Choi, E. Tello-Ruiz, I. Maricic, M. A. Bah, Y. Wu, D. Amante, D. H. Park, Y. Dia, A. R. Ali, F. I. Zaidi, A. Generotti, K. Y. Kim, T. A. Herring, S. Reeder, V. M. Andrade, K. Buttigieg, G. Zhao, J. M.

Wu, D. Li, L. Bao, J. Liu, W. Deng, C. Qin, A. S. Brown, M. Khoshnejad, N. Wang, J. Chu, D. Wrapp, J. S. McLellan, K. Muthumani, B. Wang, M. W. Carroll, J. J. Kim, J. Boyer, D. W. Kulp, Lmpf Humeau, D. B. Weiner, and K. E. Broderick. 2020. "Immunogenicity of a DNA vaccine candidate for COVID-19." *Nat Commun* 11 (1):2601. -0.

Yu, J., L. H. Tostanoski, L. Peter, N. B. Mercado, K. McMahan, S. H. Mahrokhian, J. P. Nkolola, J. Liu, Z. Li, A. Chandrashekar, D. R. Martinez, C. Loos, C. Atyeo, S. Fischinger, J. S. Burke, M. D. Slein, Y. Chen, A. Zuiani, N. Lelis FJ, M. Travers, S. Habibi, L. Pessaint, A. Van Ry, K. Blade, R. Brown, A. Cook, B. Finneyfrock, A. Dodson, E. Teow, J. Velasco, R. Zahn, F. Wegmann, E. A. Bondzie, G. Dagotto, M. S. Gebre, X. He, C. Jacob-Dolan, M. Kirilova, N. Kordana, Z. Lin, L. F. Maxfield, F. Nampanya, R. Nityanandam, J. D. Ventura, H. Wan, Y. Cai, B. Chen, A. G. Schmidt, D. R. Wesemann, R. S. Baric, G. Alter, H. Andersen, M. G. Lewis, and D. H. Barouch. 2020. "DNA vaccine protection against SARS-CoV-2 in rhesus macaques."

AFTERWORD

On December 31, 2019, the Chinese authorities recognized that a few cases of a severe lung infection might be caused by a new type of virus. Shortly after, it was established that a new type of coronavirus, the COVID-19 virus, had emerged.

At the beginning, there were only a few infected people in the city of Wuhan in China, and no COVID-19-related deaths were reported before January 9.

In mid-March, WHO declared the COVID-19 disease to be a pandemic. Shortly after, most countries started implementing lockdowns and other measures to decrease the risk of COVID-19 infections. The measures included isolation, quarantine, social distancing, school closures, flight suspensions, use of face mask, improved hand hygiene, monitoring of our movements, and many more strategies.

The measures were reasonably effective in many countries. As an example, the number of new COVID-19 cases per day in the US peaked for the first time in late April 2020, when slightly more than 32,000 new cases per day were reported.

After a few months, many countries (including the US) started to ease their lockdown measures. As a result, the number of new cases per day started to increase again. On July 2, the number of new cases in the US surpassed 53,000. Globally, the number of infection cases exceeded 11 million people. And more than 500,000 have died from the disease. The COVID-19 virus is not under control.

Lockdown measures cannot be maintained forever without causing severe damage to our societies, our economies, and our personal lives. However, as soon as the lockdown measures are eased, the number of new cases per day starts increasing again.

And as we've seen in this book (Chapter 1), it would take too long and cost too many lives to wait for immunity against the COVID-

19 virus to develop through natural infections. Our only chance of getting the pandemic under control, or even ending it, is by developing one or more effective new vaccines against the COVID-19 virus.

On May 15, 2020 (a few days after I started writing this book), WHO reported that there were eight COVID-19 vaccine candidates in clinical trials, and a further 110 candidates were under development. When I completed writing the book on June 24, there were 16 COVID-19 vaccines in clinical trials, and 125 other vaccine candidates were being developed. The 16 lead candidates have been discussed in this book.

The first results of the COVID-19 vaccine clinical trials have emerged. Some of the results were published after I completed writing this book, but before it went to press. I have to the best extent possible included the more important results of the clinical trials in this book.

The overall conclusion is that we—during the short period in which I've been writing this book—have seen tremendous progress in the development of COVID-19 vaccines and in the clinical trials of the lead candidates. Governments and big pharma companies have displayed a substantial financial and technical commitment to assisting university institutions and smaller biotech companies to develop their vaccines and to scaleup their manufacturing.

Although only a few results have been published—and no results have demonstrated that the vaccine can protect against the disease—overall the results have been encouraging. Several vaccine types have been shown to be tolerable to the test subjects and to induce good immunity against the COVID-19 virus. Regulatory authorities have shown a willingness to assist the pharma industry in quickly getting the COVID-19 vaccines to the market. This gives us hope that the first COVID-19 vaccines may already become available in 2020—at least to vaccinate the most exposed people, such as healthcare workers. Likely, billions of vaccines for mass vaccinations will not be available before 2021.

ABOUT THE AUTHOR

Dr. René Djurup graduated as a medical doctor from the University of Copenhagen in 1978. He became authorized to practice independently as a general physician in 1981. He holds a Graduate Certificate in Business Administration from Copenhagen Business School (1991) and is a certified ISO Lead Auditor.

In 1987, he received his doctoral degree from the University of Copenhagen (Doctor of Medical Sciences), based on six peer-reviewed papers in international journals.

For about nine years, Dr. Djurup worked in university hospitals in the Greater Copenhagen area, mostly within the fields of clinical immunology and allergy. In 1987, he joined the pharma company Novo (today Novo Nordisk) as a research fellow. He served Novo Nordisk for 14 years within the areas of research, development, manufacturing, quality control, and general administration.

In 2000, he co-founded the biotech company Leukotech, based on the discovery of a protein HBP that plays a key role in regulating the native immune system. He served as President and CEO of Leukotech. In this position, he filed three patent applications relating to immune modulatory peptides and the use of HBP to treat severe pneumonia. He and his team worked with the expression of recombinant proteins in the HEK293 cell lines and with chemically synthesized peptides HBP. HBP and HBP-derived peptides were tested in several animal models for infectious diseases.

In 2003, he was appointed Chief Technical Officer and Executive Vice-President of the vaccine company Bavarian Nordic. His task was to establish a vaccine manufacturing factory from scratch and to scale up the manufacturing by a factor of more than 100. The design and construction of the vaccine factory was accomplished in record time. The factory was designed to manufacture millions of doses of a safe third-generation smallpox vaccine, ordered by US governmental agencies (NIH, HHS,

BARDA). In his time at Bavarian Nordic, Dr. Djurup and his team also worked with several recombinant vaccines targeting—among others—HIV, Japanese encephalitis, and various cancers. He and his team worked with chicken embryo cells, immortalized avian cell lines, and avian stem cells. They also developed a new method for the purification of the vaccinia virus.

After he had completed his work at Bavarian Nordic, Dr. Djurup established himself as an independent consultant for vaccine development, manufacturing, and testing. He has served clients from North America, Europe, Asia, and Australia. As a consultant, he has worked with many different vaccine types including recombinant vaccines, virus-like particles, and synthetic peptide vaccines targeting malaria; hand, foot, and mouth disease (HFMD); and more. He wrote the technical documentation for the HFMD vaccine, which was used as the basis of the application for initiating clinical trials.

Dr. Djurup is the author of 39 complete peer-reviewed scientific papers and 23 congress presentations. He has filed four patent applications and holds the patent for the purification of vaccinia viruses.

He began writing compendia in 1973 as a medical student. His first university textbook, *Human Genetics*, was published in 1976. Dr. Djurup has since written 19 textbooks and popular science books about human genetics, human biochemistry, computer software, home networks, mobile computing, economics, and finance.

www.ingramcontent.com/pod-product-compliance
Lightning Source LLC
LaVergne TN
LVHW020054210726

843507LV00016B/2270